BALANCE EXERCISES FOR SENIORS OVER 60

Stay Safe and Prevent Falls with Illustrated At-Home Exercises. Increase Stability and Improve Posture with 10-Minute Daily Workouts

STEVEN MILLS

© Copyright 2022 - All rights reserved.

The content contained within this book may not be reproduced, duplicated or transmitted without direct written permission from the author or the publisher.

Under no circumstances will any blame or legal responsibility be held against the publisher, or author, for any damages, reparation, or monetary loss due to the information contained within this book, either directly or indirectly.

Legal Notice:

This book is copyright protected. It is only for personal use. You cannot amend, distribute, sell, use, quote or paraphrase any part, or the content within this book, without the consent of the author or publisher.

Disclaimer Notice:

Please note the information contained within this document is for educational and entertainment purposes only. All effort has been executed to present accurate, up to date, reliable, complete information. No warranties of any kind are declared or implied. Readers acknowledge that the author is not engaged in the rendering of legal, financial, medical or professional advice. The content within this book has been derived from various sources. Please consult a licensed professional before attempting any techniques outlined in this book.

By reading this document, the reader agrees that under no circumstances is the author responsible for any losses, direct or indirect, that are incurred as a result of the use of the information contained within this document, including, but not limited to, errors, omissions, or inaccuracies.

We invite you to scan this **QR code** using the camera of your phone to access your bonus content:

SCAN THE QR CODE BELOW

You will access to **2 EBOOKS**:

1. **"Health Tips for Seniors":** The top 10 essential life tips for seniors! These strategies will help you look and feel younger in a matter of a few weeks!

2. **"Joint Health 101":** Discover the secret to healthy joints with natural home remedies, excellent exercise tips, healthy lifestyles and more

TABLE OF CONTENTS

Introduction 14

Chapter 1: The Value of Balance 18
    The Benefits of Exercising and Improving Your Balance 19
    The Science Behind Physical Balance. 21
        How Often Should Seniors Do Balance Exercises? 22
        General Tips for Finding Your Balance. 22

Chapter 2: Exercising Safely 24
    How to Exercise Safely. 25
    Chronic Conditions and Impairments. 26
        Alzheimer's Disease and Related Cognitive Impairments. 26
        Arthritis 27
        Osteoporosis. 27
        Chronic Obstructive Pulmonary Disease 27
        Type 2 Diabetes 27
        Overweight 28
    Exercises to Avoid. 28

Chapter 3: Warming Up 30
    Warm Up Exercises 31
        Beginner Level 31
            Head Rotations 31
            Shoulder Rolls 32
            Single Leg Stance 33
            Single Leg Stance With an Arm 34
        Intermediate Level 35

    Balancing Wand..35

    Tree Pose..36

    Single Leg Raise..37

    Heel-To-Toe Walking.......................................38

  Advanced Level..39

    Sit-To-Stand...39

    Upper Body Rotations.....................................40

    Testing Your Balance.....................................41

Chapter 4: Seated Exercises.....................................42

  Ten Exercises That You Can Do While Sitting....................43

  Stretching Exercises..44

    Beginner Stretches.......................................44

      Seated Backbend.....................................44

      Seated Overhead Stretch.............................45

      Seated Hip Stretch..................................46

    Medium Level Stretch....................................47

      Seated Side Stretch.................................47

  Chair Exercises..48

    Easy Chair Exercises.....................................48

      Chair Leg Raises....................................48

      Seated Knee-to-Chest................................49

      Knee Extensions.....................................50

      Heel Slides...51

      Seated Calf Raises..................................52

    Medium to Advanced Chair Exercises......................53

      Seated Extended Leg Raises..........................53

      Leg Kicks...54

      Variations of Seated Exercises......................55

  Seated Knee-to-Chest Variation..55

  Seated Extended Leg Raises..56

Chapter 5: Standing Exercises 58

 Ten Exercises That You Can Do While Standing 59

  Easy Standing Exercises 60

   Calf Stretch..60

   Ladder.. 61

   Toe Lifts...62

   Marching on the Spot...63

  Medium Standing Exercises 64

   Rock the Boat..64

   Side-Step Walk...65

   Stepping Stones 66

   Step Ups 67

   Standing Back Leg Raises...68

   Side Leg Raises..69

Chapter 6: Walking Exercises 70

 Ten Exercises That You Can Do While Walking 73

  Easy Walking Exercises.. 74

   Marching On The Spot with Arms 74

   Side-to-Side Taps 75

   Lateral Step 76

   Heel Touches... 77

   Heel-to-Toe Touches.. 78

  Medium Walking Exercises.. 79

   Knee Ups 79

   Zig-Zag Walking..80

  Obstacles 81

 Advanced Walking Exercises 82

  Step-Ups at a Faster Pace 82

  Aerobic Challenge 83

Chapter 7: Targeting Specific Areas of the Body 84

 Leg Stengthening Exercises 85

  Easy Leg Strengthing Exercises. 86

   Hip Extensions 86

   Lunges. 87

  Medium to Advanced Leg Strengthing Exercises. 88

   Reverse Lunges. 88

   Modified Squats. 89

   Single Leg Cross-Body Punches 90

 Core Strengthing Exercises 91

  Easy Core Strengthining Exercises 92

   Seated Half Roll-Backs. 92

   Seated Forward Roll-Ups. 93

   Seated Side Bends 94

  Medium to Advanced Core Strengthing Exercises. 95

   Superman 95

   Modified Planks 96

 Upper Body Strengthening Exercises 97

  Easy Upper Body Strengthening Exercises. 98

   Bicep Curls 98

   Triceps Kickbacks 99

  Medium to Advanced Upper Body Strengthening Exercises. 100

   Diagonal Inward Shoulder Raise 100

   Diagonal Outward Shoulder Raise. 101

      Overhead Press. 102

   Stretching Exercises. 103

      Neck Stretch. 104

      Shoulder and Upper Arm Stretch. 105

      Quadriceps Stretch. 106

      Hip Stretch 107

      Lower Back Stretch. 108

Chapter 8: Vestibular Exercises 110

   Exercises to Improve Your Vestibular Organ 113

      Head Exercises. 113

      Turning Side to Side. 114

      Standing and Throwing a Ball. 115

      Walking While Turning Your Head 116

      Lying Down 117

      Gaze Stabilization. 118

Chapter 9: Exercising With a Partner 120

   Safety Notes When Exercising With a Partner 122

   Exercises You Can Do With a Partner. 123

      Back Rows with a Resistance Band 123

      Neck Exercise 124

      Partner Pushes. 125

      Partner Pulls 126

   Other Fun Activities to Do With a Partner. 127

      Dancing. 127

      Playing Catch or Frisbee 127

Chapter 10: Exercises with Equipment...........................128

Five Exercise Ball Exercises...129
Benefits of Medicine Balls..129
Tummy Twists...130
Circle Press..131
Thigh Squeeze..132
Seated Ball Balance..133
Hip Lifts...134

Five Resistance Band Exercises......................................135
Benefits of Using Resistance Bands............................135
External Rotation..136
Bent Over Pulldowns..137
Leg Extension..138
Standing Adduction...139
Lateral Band Walk..140

Five Dumbell Exercises..141
Benefits of Using Dumbells.....................................141
Front Raise..142
Triceps Extensions...143
Dumbbell Lunge...144
One Legged Deadlift..145
Romanian Lunge...146

Five Balance Pad Exercises...147
Benefits of Using Balance Pads.................................147
Side-to-Side Steps...148
Marching in Place..149
Single Leg Balance...150
Squats...151
Front Elevated Lunge.......................................152

Chapter 11: Weekly Workout Planner 154

  Workout Plans You Can Follow 155

    Beginner Level Workout Plan 155

      Monday 155

      Tuesday 155

      Wednesday 156

      Thursday 156

      Friday 156

      Saturday 156

      Sunday 157

    Medium Level Workout Plan 157

      Monday 157

      Tuesday 157

      Wednesday 157

      Thursday 158

      Friday 158

      Saturday 158

      Sunday 158

    Advanced Level Workout Plan 159

      Monday 159

      Tuesday 159

      Wednesday 159

      Thursday 160

      Friday 160

      Saturday 160

      Sunday 160

    Stretching Morning and Night Routines 161

      Monday to Sunday Mornings 161

      Monday to Sunday Evenings 161

    Ten Minute Routines... 162
        Monday, Wednesday, and Friday 162
        Tuesday, Thursday, Saturday.. 162
        Sunday 162

Conclusion **163**

Glossary **164**

References **165**

INTRODUCTION

Being balanced is the ability to feel steady and stable while you are seated or standing. Having a good balance means you can easily control your body's position while performing daily activities such as standing, using the stairs, and walking. However, when a fall happens, it is usually due to your balance getting lost, and your insufficient ability to regain your balance.

Several conditions can be the root of the issue for seniors who struggle to maintain balance. For example, you likely feel like your ups and downs are not correct, or you feel unsteady on your feet, which may result in falling. But what if this feeling of being unbalanced is new to you? In that case, several things may be causing it, such as medication or a heart condition. It may even result from social, economic, behavioral, or environmental factors.

If you feel this new unsteady feeling is persistent, or leaves you lightheaded, dizzy, shakey, or unstable, it is recommended that you talk to your physician. There is hope, though, as some conditions can be reversed with the help of your doctor and some basic exercises.

How do our bodies balance, though? Our bodies have systems that work together to maintain balance in an upright position. This includes:

- Your vision
- Your vestibular system (located in your inner ear)
- The nerves throughout your body that communicate to your brain where your body is in space
- Your cerebellum, the brain's balance center

- Your brain which processes information given to send the right messages to your body
- Your muscles and nerves functioning to receive the messages sent by the brain

Regardless of the length of time you may have dealt with feeling dizzy, you likely have found it challenging to maintain a stable, upright position. In addition, feeling unbalanced might be impacting your ability to carry out daily tasks like getting dressed, eating and cooking, bathing, or moving around your home. Additionally, the balance issues you may be dealing with now will likely worsen as you age. This is not meant to alarm you, of course, but to bring your awareness to that possibility, if not your current reality.

Today, those aged 65 and up commonly visit their doctors when balance issues arise. So, naturally, it is understandable to feel worried when you can no longer trust that you will remain upright. Additionally, risks and injuries rise when you begin to have balance issues. Some of these issues can include a heart condition, or a problem in your brain or nervous system. Regardless of the circumstances, check in with your healthcare provider to identify the root of the balance issue and recommended treatments.

However, there are some things you can do outside of the medications prescribed by your doctor, that can also help with your balance issues. This book will give you some balance exercises at various levels to improve your ability to maintain control and stability of your body. This book will teach you:

- The science of physical balance and the factors that lead to poor balance
- How often you should do the exercises and tips on finding your balance
- How to exercise safely
- The importance of warming up
- Seated exercises you can do while watching television and their benefits

- Exercises you can do standing and their benefits
- Walking exercises
- Focusing on areas that are important to maintain balance
- Vestibular exercises, and when you might need to use these
- Exercising with a partner
- Using equipment for balance exercising

Additionally, this book will provide the facts and information you need to feel confident in the exercises and yourself. You will also gain the knowledge and understand the benefits of each exercise outlined in the book. Each exercise is designed to help you strengthen the muscles to help you stay upright and stable on your feet. Working on specific muscle groups, like your legs and core, will help reduce the risk of falling. You will find that your balance will improve with the various exercises outlined in each chapter. After reading this and trying out the exercises yourself, over time you should be able to:

- Hold a position for longer
- Add movement to the position
- Close your eyes and maintain your balance
- Be able to remove supporting equipment such as a chair

How can you trust that these exercises will improve your confidence, though? Well, a study done on 104 elderly adults in Nakhon Si Thammarat Province, Thailand, showed an improvement in their balance after three months of training. In addition, the participants found that their fear of falling had reduced at the three-, six-, nine-, and twelve-month marks. So if this group of adults can feel empowered to take control of their balance, you can too!

Falling is one of the major reasons injury and death happens in seniors. It is estimated that about 40% of seniors aged 65 and over will fall at least once; one in three adults who are 65 will be affected annually. Other studies suggest about 50 to 60% of falls happen within the home due to clutter, lack of railings along stairs, loose rugs, no grab bars in the bathroom, or poor lighting. These falls often result in serious injury such as broken bones or serious concussions, or sometimes, sadly, they are fatal. You can understand the importance of working on balance skills to prepare you in the event you trip.

CHAPTER ONE
THE VALUE OF BALANCE

When we were young, we learned to build our balance skill set through various activities like jumping, climbing (whether a tree or playground equipment), walking along walls or train tracks, and spinning. As we get older, though, we tend to forget the value of balance, and therefore take it for granted.

When our systems are healthily balanced, we feel more energized and robust, allowing us to move through our day quickly and with total confidence. Keeping our system in check and healthy is essential, especially if you have joint pain, a weak skeletal system, or are easily dizzy.

Interestingly, our balance begins to decrease when we hit the age of 35, but you likely didn't notice at the time unless you had an issue with your sense of balance due to vertigo or dizziness. It could have been a sign that something is wrong with your vestibular system, such as Meniere's Disease, in which case you would want to seek treatment from your physician. Other contributing factors to balance issues alongside old age may be overlooked, such as a decrease or loss in sight, loss of musculoskeletal strength, cognitive impairment, or a B12 deficiency. These factors can directly impact you, and make you feel unsteady on your feet, which is why the risk of falling increases as you age.

THE BENEFITS OF EXERCISING AND IMPROVING YOUR BALANCE

One of the contributing factors to a decline in our balance system is our proprioception, which can worsen as we age. By doing balance exercises, you will reduce the risk of injury, and avoid fatal risks.

Having balance issues can be compared to spraining an ankle. Once you sprain your ankle, you are at risk for re-injury unless you take the necessary steps to rehab it to retrain the balance. When a sprained ankle occurs, the muscles stabilizing the joint stop working together, destabilizing the ankle joint. Balancing exercises following the injury help rebuild the muscle to contract and support the ankle joint during activities; it can also help prevent re-injuring it.

Why do most seniors fall at some point? These are some of the reasons why you might lose balance:

- A deterioration in your vision prevents you from seeing clearly
- Poor posture, osteoporosis, or spinal degeneration makes it difficult to stand straight
- A weakness in your legs or hips makes it harder to walk
- Lifting our feet as we walk can get more challenging, which leads to stumbling or tripping
- A decrease in reaction when something is in our pathway
- Taking medications that can make you feel lightheaded, dizzy, or drowsy
- Low blood pressure

Here are some of the other benefits of exercising to help you with your balance:

- Your independence will improve because your muscles and endurance will strengthen, decreasing your fall risk
- Your immune system will improve
- A better digestive system will result
- You will have better blood circulation and pressure, reducing the risk of a stroke or heart attack
- You will have a decreased chance of getting diabetes, or if you do have diabetes, exercise will help control it
- Bone density will improve and reduce the risk of broken bones
- It will help prevent Alzheimer's Disease
- There will be weight-loss opportunities
- There will be decreased chance of getting heart disease
- You will have a reduced chance of developing osteoporosis

THE SCIENCE BEHIND PHYSICAL BALANCE

We know our balance is working well when we do the following activities without issue:

- Getting out of bed
- Getting in or out of a chair
- Going up or down the stairs
- Walking outside on an uneven pathway

Our brain, nervous system, muscles, and bones need to work together to prevent us from falling. Balance and equilibrium are controlled by the messages our brain sends to our eyes, inner ear, muscle joints, and other sensory systems. Together, they make up the vestibular system.

Inside our ears are three semicircular canals with fluid and sensors to detect how our head is moving. When our heads turn in one direction, the hair cells in the canals will send nerve signals to the brain. The brain then takes the nerve signals and processes them to help us know if we are in a space, like a room, or if we are moving, like walking. When we are not receiving the correct sensory information from our eyes, tendons, muscles, joints, and balance organs in our inner ears, our brain stem cannot process the information to help you understand your surroundings, or if you are moving.

How Often Should Seniors Do Balance Exercises?

The Center for Disease Control and Prevention (2019) suggests that adults who are 65 and over should practice balance exercises at least three times a week. They also recommend adults in this age category be active for at least "150 minutes a week of moderate-intensity exercises," or "75 minutes of vigorous-intensity activities" (Center for Disease Control and Prevention, 2019). Your workout routine could look like this:

- Do a moderate-intensity aerobic workout such as walking for 30 minutes five times a week. In addition, you would want to include muscle strengthening to work all of your major muscle groups (arms, shoulders, chest, back, abdomen, legs, and hips) and balance activity.

- For a vigorous-intensity routine, jog, run, or hike for 75 minutes weekly alongside muscle strengthening and balance activities.

- Do a mix between the two on two or more days a week, combined with strength and balance training

General Tips for Finding Your Balance

Here are some tips to get you started on helping you maintain and improve your balance as you move through this book:

- Make sure to use your hips! Our lumbopelvic complex contributes to our overall body balance. When you continue to work on your core and hip strength, the muscles in this area will help you feel more stable on your feet.

- Make sure to stand while exercising as long as you feel comfortable. For example, you could stand while doing bicep curls or overhead presses.
- Continue to practice getting in and out of seated positions, and on and off the floor.
- Try to stand on one leg for 10 seconds, then switch to the other leg.

CHAPTER TWO
EXERCISING SAFELY

Exercising safely is essential to any fitness routine or program to get the most out of your workouts. Any information regarding exercises and safety should always be given to you by your physician, sports medicine doctor, physiotherapist, occupational therapist, or exercise physiologist. Safety while you exercise needs to be a priority over everything else, to prevent getting hurt while you workout.

While performing any exercise, be mindful if the activity or technique is safe based on if you have a pre-existing injury, or your current fitness level. Existing injuries need to rest. When you try to push through the pain, you risk worsening the injury ,and delaying the healing. Also, remember that any exercise will always pose a risk of injury. If at any point you feel discomfort, it's best to modify or avoid specific activities. However, if your body is signaling fatigue or pain, stop. Further into this chapter, you will learn about some exercises you should avoid trying. You should also stop exercising and seek medical attention if you have discomfort or pain in your chest, have trouble catching your breath, or are experiencing irregular or a very fast heartbeat. Lastly, it's also essential to avoid doing the same daily routine, and work to have at least one or two recovery days in the week.

HOW TO EXERCISE SAFELY

When you are learning how to do an exercise, it's essential to follow the instructions on how to do it. Although modifying a movement might be necessary, avoid changing the exercise altogether, as it can increase your risk of injury.

For clothing, make sure you are wearing clothes that fit you well. Avoid wearing baggy or tight clothing, and uncomfortable shoes.

You should also be aware of your surroundings. For example, if you struggle with hearing, have a workout partner to help prevent you from bumping into something that could make you fall. Risks of falling can also be increased if you have other issues such as poor vision, memory problems, and a cognitive decline, all of which can be assisted by a partner.

It is also vital to remain hydrated while exercising, to reduce the risk of becoming lightheaded, dizzy, or faint.

To have an effective and safe workout, warm up at least 5-10 minutes before beginning to activate your muscles. Different warm-up exercises you can do will be elaborated upon in the next chapter.

CHRONIC CONDITIONS AND IMPAIRMENTS

It's no secret that our ticking heart is what keeps everything else in our bodies functioning. As we age, we experience changes in the heart and blood vessels, which is normal! However, some changes can occur due to disease too. Inactive people are likelier to develop heart disease compared to active ones.

Even if you have a pre-existing health condition, you can still exercise. Chronic pain can be reduced when you exercise. If you remain inactive, the risks of more pain and loss of function can increase.

Keep in mind that inflammation, pain, or swelling can happen when you exercise. When it does, make sure to focus on different areas for a day or two, to allow your body to recover.

Alzheimer's Disease and Related Cognitive Impairments

Exercise may help slow down mild cognitive impairment in older adults. Exercise can also help an older adult's overall brain function, especially for those at risk for Alzheimer's Disease. People living with Alzheimer's or a different form of dementia can feel good, and maintain a healthy weight, by remaining active.

For caregivers taking care of their elderly parents living with Alzheimer's, there are options to make exercise fun too!

Here are some exercise ideas for people living with cognitive issues:
- Take a walk with a partner or a caregiver
- Use exercise videos from platforms such as YouTube
- Dance it out

If you have difficulty walking, try using a stationary bike, a soft ball to toss back and forth, stretching bands, or household items for light weight-lifting.

Arthritis

Exercise can help reduce the pain, stiffness, and stress on your joints in combination with losing weight. With arthritis, you can try flexibility exercises such as Tai Chi, strengthening exercises such as overhead arm raises, resistance bands, or endurance exercises like swimming.

Osteoporosis

By doing activities such as walking, jogging, or dancing, you are forced to work against gravity, allowing you to build your muscles and strengthen bones if you struggle with osteoporosis.

Chronic Obstructive Pulmonary Disease

If you have chronic obstructive pulmonary disease, it's best to talk with your pulmonary therapist to see what exercises they recommend. The rehabilitation programs will help you learn to exercise while managing the disease.

Type 2 Diabetes

A regular exercise routine will help manage the disease and give you longevity. For example, taking a walk every day helps manage your glucose levels. So here is a challenge: set a goal to remain active throughout the week, such as a moderate-aerobic workout for 30 minutes at least five times a week, combined with strength and a balance exercises.

Also, try stretching between commercial breaks or while streaming a program. You can also walk around while talking on the phone. If you are running errands, try parking further away from the store to get in your steps.

Overweight

If you are overweight, do not get discouraged! Even if you have difficulty bending over or walking, try something like water aerobics, or dancing. Anything that will get you moving, even for a few minutes daily, is a start.

As always, seek medical or physiotherapist advice if something does not feel right.

Exercises to Avoid

The following exercises should be avoided:

Standing toe-touches.

You risk overstretching your hamstrings and lower back muscles by bending down to touch your toes with straight legs. In this move, you also risk stressing your vertebrae, discs, and muscles. Here are some alternative ideas for this exercise that you can do:

1. Place your foot on a low bench or a chair to stretch your hamstring and lower back muscles. Make sure to keep your knees soft. Reach forward gently with your arms outstretched, keeping your back straight.
2. Alternatively, you can lie down on your back on the floor to stretch your hamstrings. Keeping one leg bent, straighten one of your legs as you lift it toward the ceiling. Interlock your fingers behind your leg to support and hold for a few counts before switching to your other leg. Remember to keep your extended leg soft at the knees.
3. Sitting on the floor cross-legged, slowly lean forward with your arms stretched out. Make sure your back remains straight as you bend at your hips.

Full squats.

Performing a full squat is when you bend your knees past 90 degrees. This exercise can strain your ligaments, muscles, and cartilage around your knee joint and lower back, whether or not you are using weights. Alternatively, you can try this:

1. Try a half squat where your knees are bent at 45 degrees.
2. Use a mirror to check your form if you are going to squat to 90 degrees, or use a partner for this exercise to spot you.

Double leg raises. This exercise is done on your back with both legs lifting together. The move can add too much stress to your lower back. Here is what you can do instead:

1. Keep one leg bent with your foot on the floor.
2. Lift your other leg, and then switch. Ensure to keep your hips stable throughout the movement.

Sit-ups.

Two variations can cause you injury doing sit-ups. One of the ways you can become injured is by having a partner anchor your feet to the floor. The second way you can be injured is by keeping your legs straight. Also, having your hands clasped behind your head or neck while your body is moving can cause strain to your lower back. As a variation to a sit-up, try doing abdominal curls instead:

1. Lie down on your back with your knees and feet drawn in a comfortable position. Your feet should be flat on the floor.
2. Cross your arms over your chest to make an X or keep them alongside your torso.
3. As you breathe, curl your spine to bring your rib cage toward your pelvis.
4. Inhale and uncurl to return to the starting position.

CHAPTER THREE
WARMING UP

Warming up before your workout helps to enlarge your blood vessels to ensure your muscles get enough oxygen while you exercise. Warm-ups also help raise your muscles' temperature to optimize flexibility, while reducing stress on your heart. Fatty acids and carbohydrates will also be converted to energy when hormones release.

The recommended time to do warm-ups is between five and ten minutes. The more intense your workout, the longer your warm-up should be. Make sure to move slowly and use your entire body. Let's take a look at a variety of warm-up exercises you can do. These exercises will be listed from beginner level to more experienced.

WARM UP EXERCISES- BEGINNER LEVEL

HEAD ROTATIONS

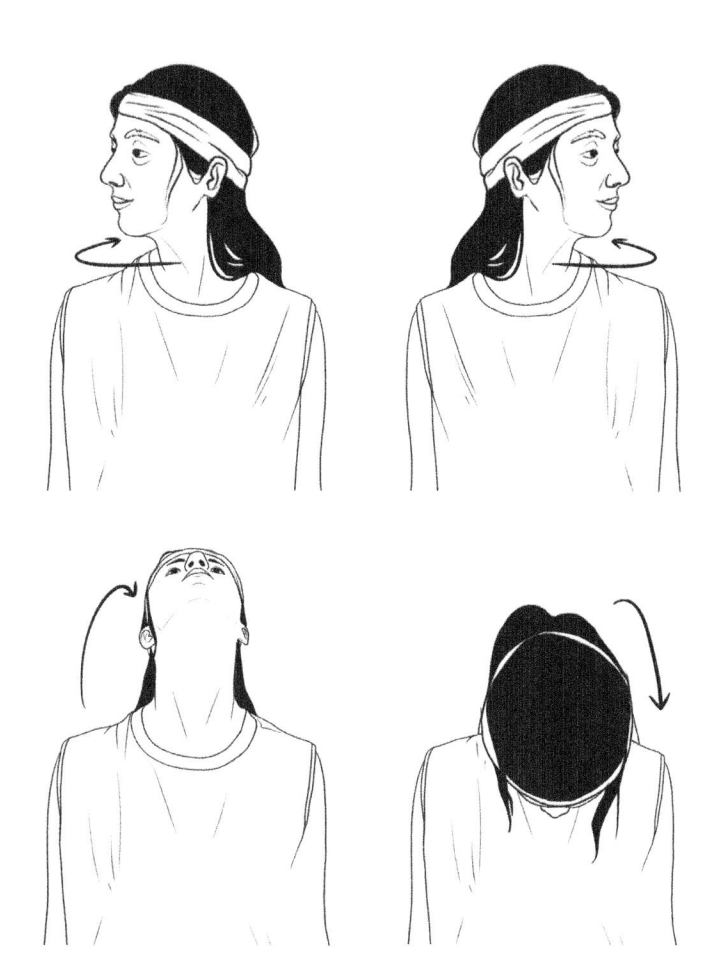

INTRODUCTION

Doing head rotations helps improve your balance and strengthen your neck muscles. Head rotations can be done seated or standing.

INSTRUCTIONS

1. Standing or sitting tall, turn your head from left to right slowly.
2. After that, nod your head up and down to complete an entire circuit.
3. Repeat in the opposite direction.

Complete 5-10 repetitions.

WARM UP EXERCISES- BEGINNER LEVEL

SHOULDER ROLLS

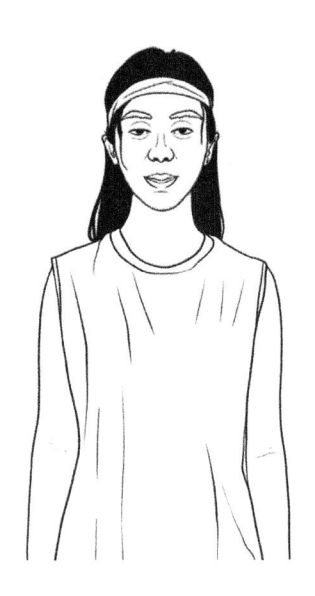

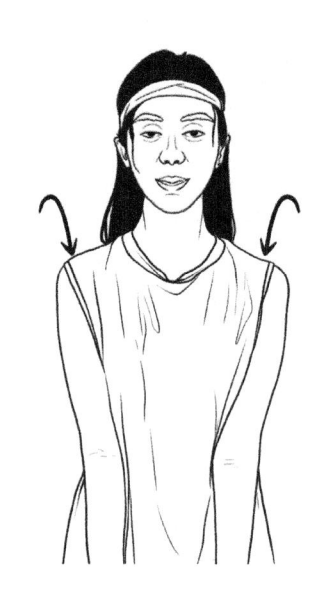

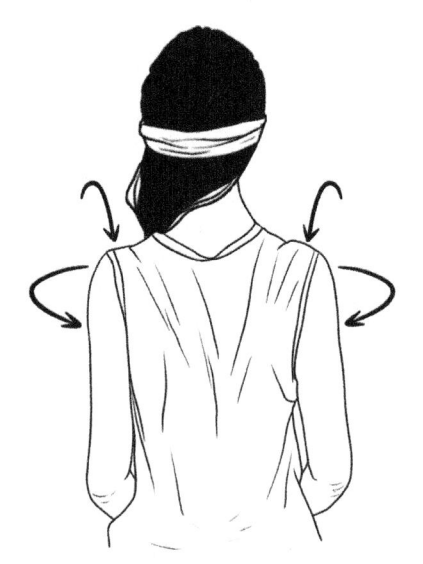

INTRODUCTION

This warm-up exercise helps improve your arm mobility and core strength. Shoulder rolls can be done standing or sitting.

INSTRUCTIONS

1. Bring your shoulders up to your ears, and rotate them to the back, bringing your
2. shoulder blades down to open your chest.
3. Repeat this motion for 5-10 repetitions.

Next you will reverse your shoulder rolls to go forward.

As you did before, bring your shoulders to your ears, and roll your shoulders forward.

Reset by pulling your shoulder blades down to open your chest.

Repeat the motion for 5-10 repetitions.

For a variation, try bending your elbows to create chicken wings as you roll your shoulders backward and forward.

WARM UP EXERCISES- BEGINNER LEVEL

SINGLE LEG STANCE

INTRODUCTION

The single leg stance helps strengthen your core. Use the back of a chair, table, or countertop for support.

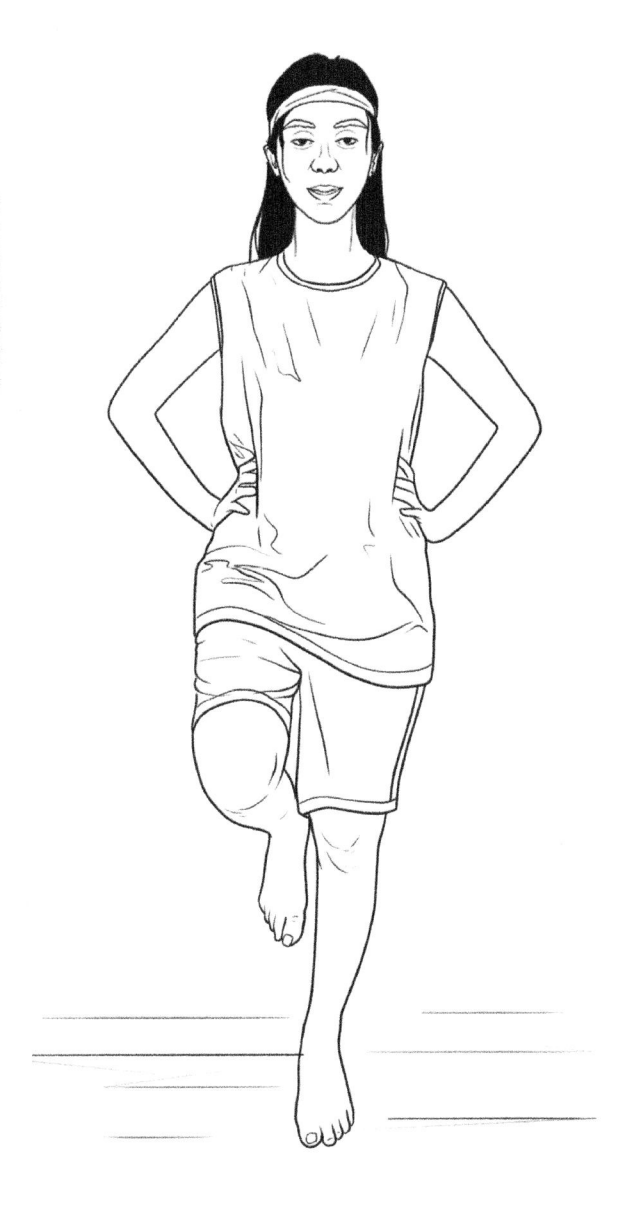

INSTRUCTIONS

1. Stand comfortably on the floor.
2. Bend your right knee, and slowly lift your right foot off the floor in front of you.
3. Hold for 10 seconds.
4. Lower it back to the floor, and switch to repeating the exercise on your left leg.

Do each cycle five or ten times on each leg.

WARM UP EXERCISES- BEGINNER LEVEL

SINGLE LEG STANCE WITH AN ARM

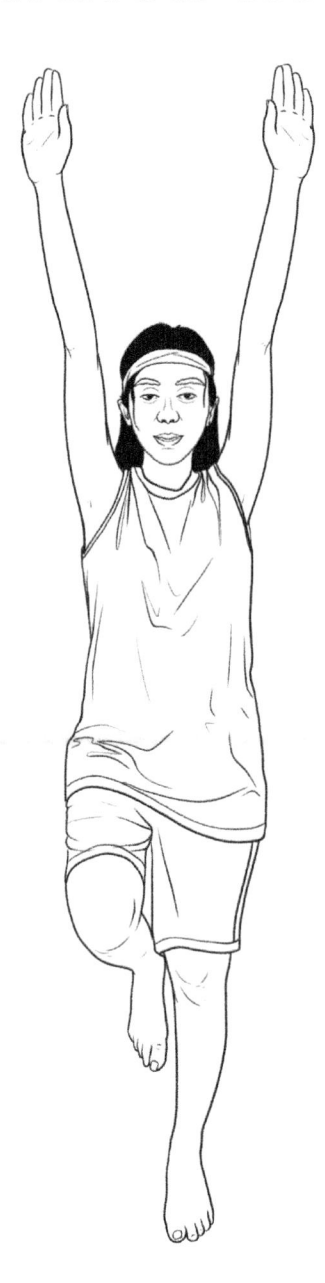

INTRODUCTION

The single leg stance with an arm adds a challenge to engage your core muscles further. Repeat the same steps from the single leg stance, except that you will simultaneously lift your arm above your head as you lift your leg. Hold for 10 seconds before lowering your foot and arm. Repeat with your left leg. To complete the cycle, repeat each leg five or ten times.

WARM UP EXERCISES- INTERMEDIATE LEVEL
BALANCING WAND

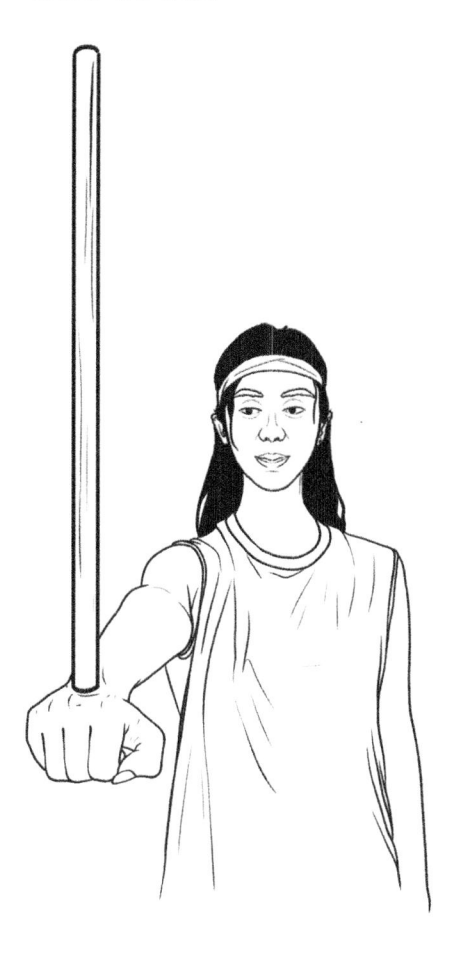

INTRODUCTION

For the balancing wand warm-up exercise, you will need a cane, an umbrella, or a broomstick. This exercise is great to help improve your balance, because it will help stabilize your center of gravity, and your hand-eye coordination.

INSTRUCTIONS

1. Sitting on a chair, hold out your non-dominant hand in front of your torso, with your palm up towards the ceiling.
2. Using your dominant hand, place the long object into your outstretched hand, and work to balance it for as long as possible.
3. Switch to the other side, repeating the exercise for 5-10 repetitions with each hand.

WARM UP EXERCISES- INTERMEDIATE LEVEL

TREE POSE

INTRODUCTION

This warm-up move is used in yoga exercises, but it challenges you to find your center of gravity while you stand on one leg. Think of it as a step up from the single leg stance, and single leg stance with an arm.

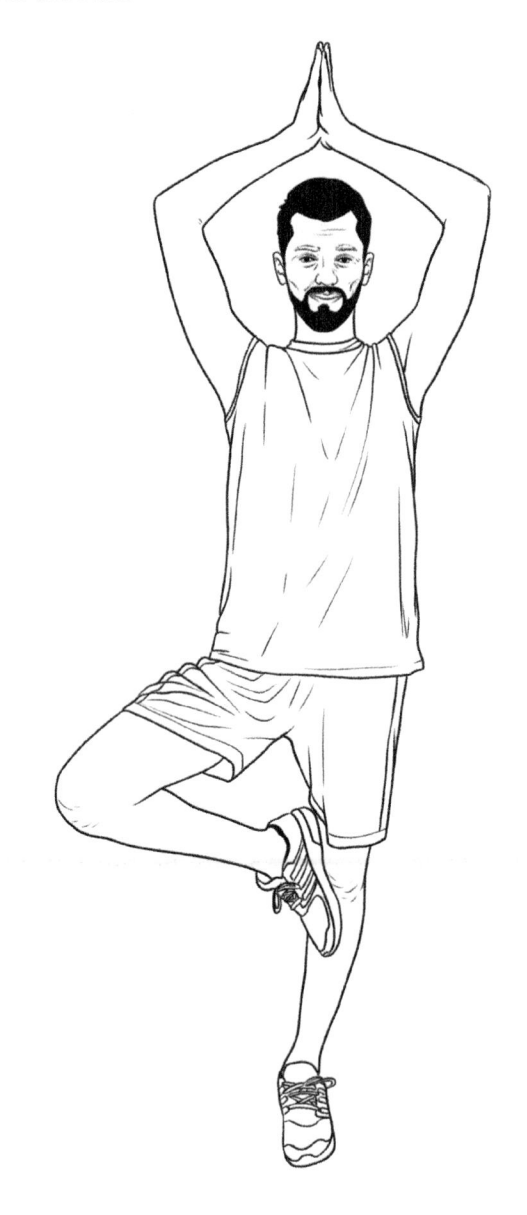

INSTRUCTIONS

1. Standing on both feet to start, transfer your weight to your right leg while you begin to raise your left foot to rest just above your ankle, with your left hip open.
2. Your knee should be facing the left side of the room.
3. Bring your palms to a prayer pose in front of you. For an added challenge, try lifting your hands above your head.
4. Try to stay in this position for a minute before lowering your left foot.

↻ Repeat on the other side.
One trick to try and keep your balance is to find a spot on the wall to focus on.

WARM UP EXERCISES- INTERMEDIATE LEVEL

SINGLE LEG RAISE

INTRODUCTION

Use the back of a chair for support while trying this balancing warm-up.

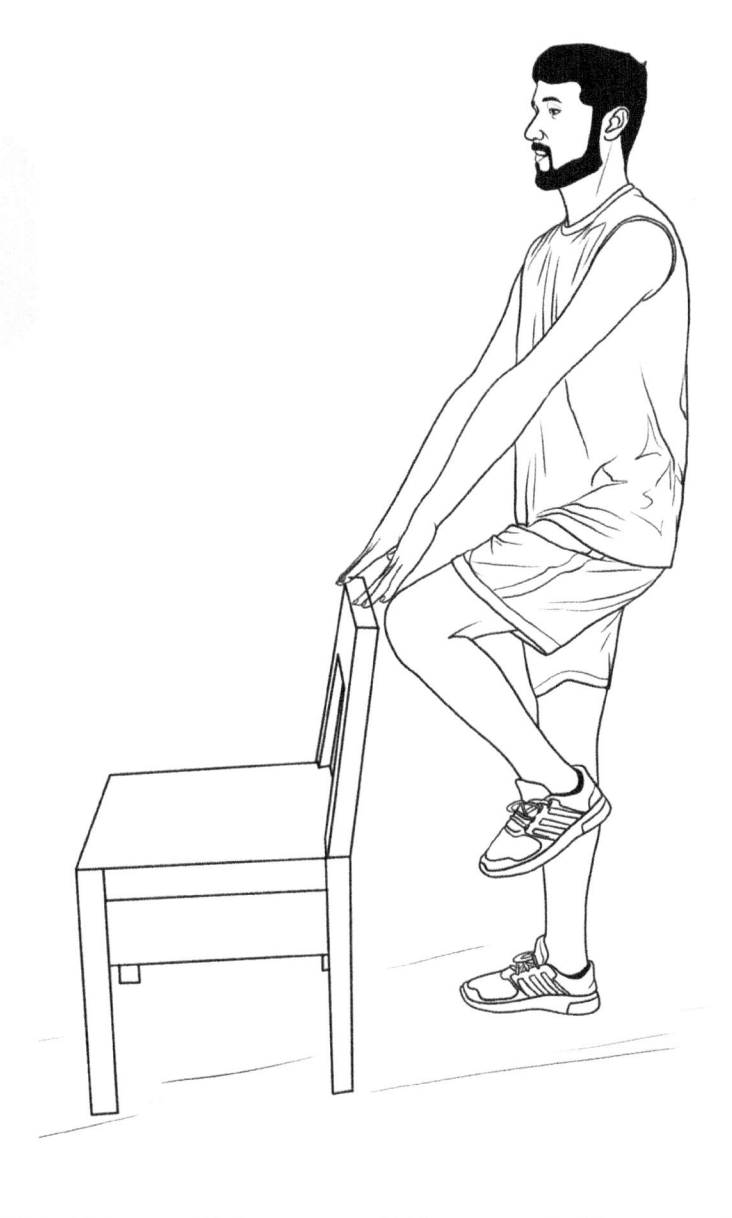

INSTRUCTIONS

1. Standing tall with your spine lengthened, lift your right foot about an inch above the ground.
2. Flex your calves by pulling your toes toward your shin for a challenge.
3. Hold for 10 seconds, and then lower your foot.
4. Repeat on the left side.

Complete this exercise five times on both sides.

WARM UP EXERCISES- INTERMEDIATE LEVEL

HEEL-TO-TOE WALKING

INTRODUCTION

For this exercise, use some imagination to make it fun, and imagine you are walking along a balance beam. This warm-up exercise activates your core muscles, while strengthening your calf muscles.

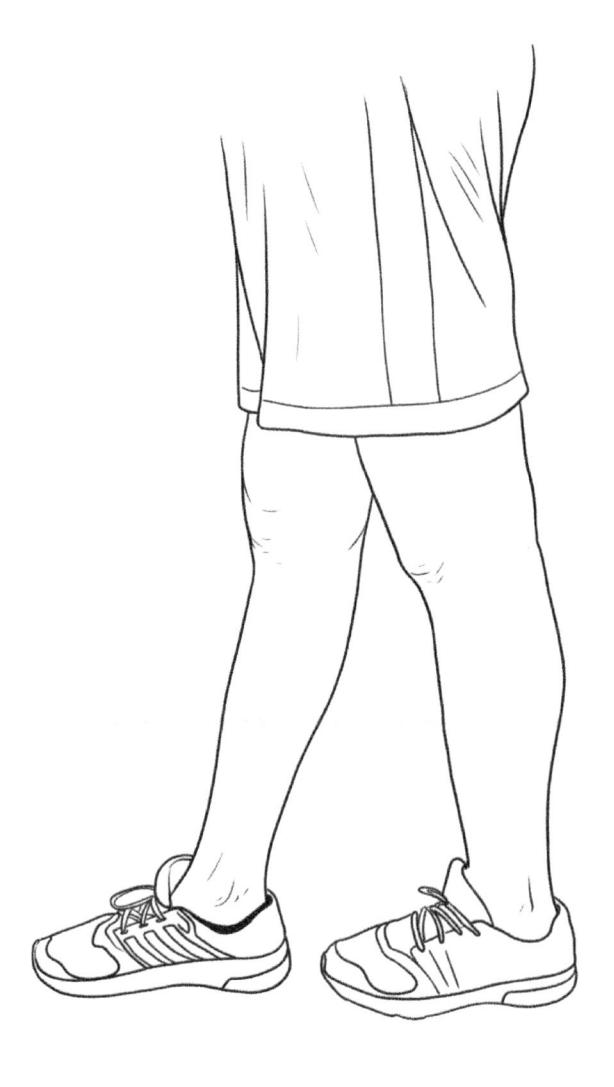

INSTRUCTIONS

1. Beginning on one side of the room, step forward with your right foot.
2. Next, step forward with your left foot, placing it directly in front of your right foot, ensuring your left heel is touching the toes of your right foot. Next, shift to place your right foot in front of your left as you did before. Take about 20 to 30 steps across the room.
3. If you find balance tricky on this one, try extending your arms out into a 'T' position to help you balance.

WARM UP EXERCISES- ADVANCED LEVEL
SIT-TO-STAND

INTRODUCTION

This warm-up exercise is good for warming up your hip flexors and lower body strength.

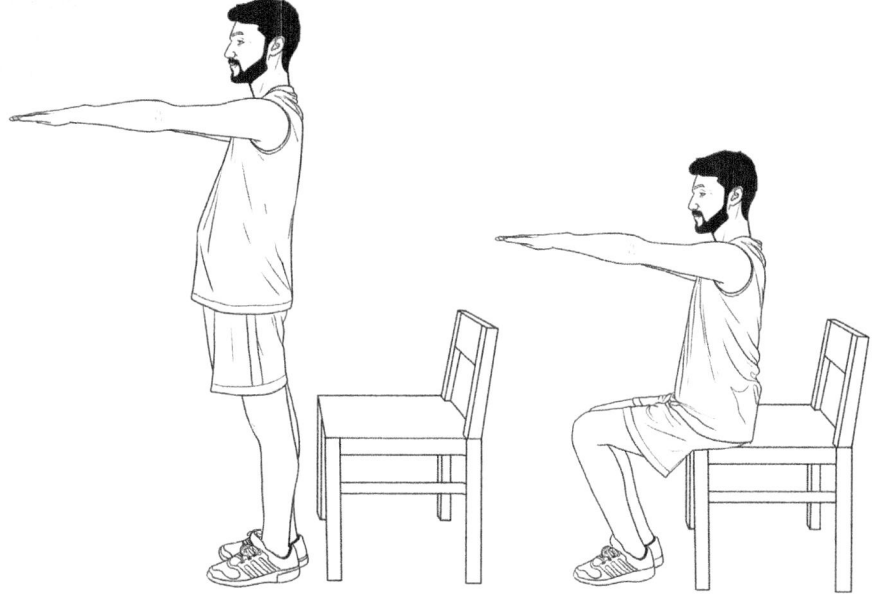

INSTRUCTIONS

1. Begin by sitting in your chair. For this exercise, it does not matter if the chair has arms. However, arms are a great support if this is a daily task you have trouble with.
2. Slowly move into a standing position to regain your balance and posture.
3. Begin to lower back down to your chair in a controlled motion. If you are using a chair with arms for support, make sure to grab the arms for support as you move closer to the chair seat.

Repeat 10-15 times.

If you are using a chair that does not have arms, it is strongly encouraged to use a cane for support. The goal here is to have you get in and out of a chair without support as you practice over time.

WARM UP EXERCISES- ADVANCED LEVEL

UPPER BODY ROTATIONS

INTRODUCTION

The upper body rotation warm-up helps build on your hip mobility and coordination.

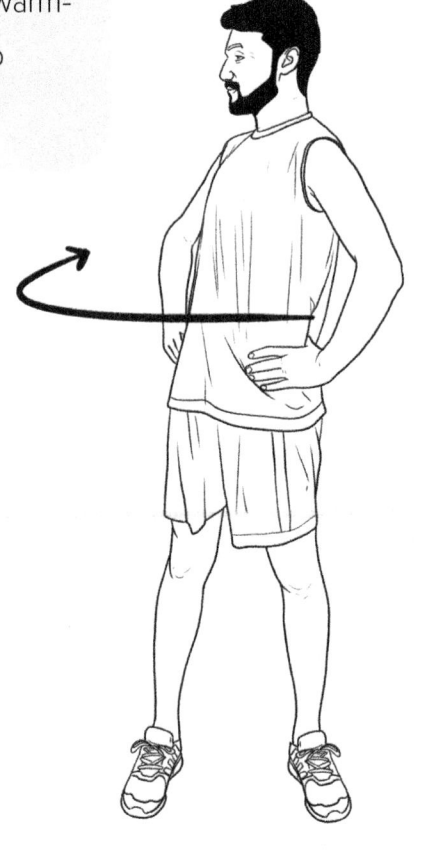

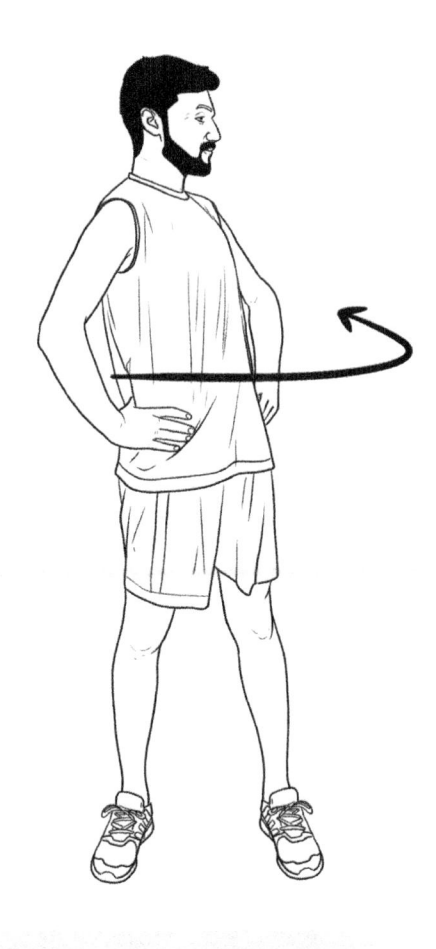

INSTRUCTIONS

1. Stand with a tall spine and place your hands on your hips.
2. Slightly bend at your hips to lean your upper body forward.
3. Push your right hip out to the side. Your left side will create a slight curve or backward 'C.'
4. Rotate your left hip forward to have a slight upper body back bend.
5. Push your left hip out to create that same slight curve on the right side.
6. Push your right hip back to bring you to the center, completing a full circle.

↻ For this rotation exercise, draw out ten circles (five in each direction).

TESTING YOUR BALANCE

If you are unsure of where your balance stands, try out these four different tests to determine your level. With each balance test, you should be able to hold the position for at least 20 to 30 seconds each, without wobbling or losing your balance.

1. Start by standing with your feet touching together. Close your eyes and stand for 30 seconds.
2. Next, you are going to stand in a tandem position. Place your left foot in front of your right (just as you tried in the heel-to-toe walk), and then close your eyes again. This might seem simple, but many have difficulty with this stance when they have poor balance.
3. Return to standing straight with your feet under your knees and hips. Lift one leg up and close your eyes.
4. Next, with your eyes remaining closed, try reaching forward as far as you can. You should be able to confidently reach at least 10 inches in front of you.

CHAPTER FOUR
SEATED EXERCISES

This chapter will walk you through various exercises you can do while sitting, watching television or waiting for your meal to be ready. These exercises are low-impact, which can be helpful to your joints. However, make sure you talk with your doctor before you begin any workout if any of the following apply to you:

New injuries that could be agitated

Recently had surgery

You find it difficult to perform the exercises due to posture issues

TEN EXERCISES THAT YOU CAN DO WHILE SITTING

For each of the following exercises, you should complete them two to three times with 8-12 repetitions, unless noted otherwise.

Before you begin the exercises, the first few are good stretching movements to warm your body further, and work on your balance while seated. These exercises can also be done while watching television.

STRETCHING EXERCISES- BEGINNER STRETCHES

SEATED BACKBEND

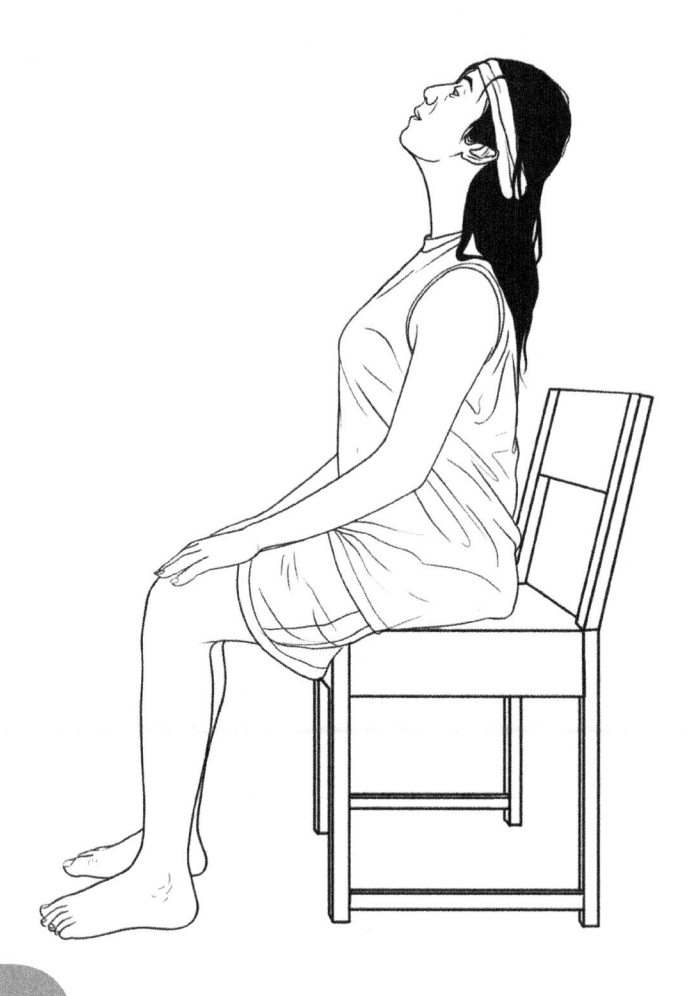

INSTRUCTIONS

1. Sit comfortably in your chair close to the edge. Sit straight to lengthen your spine to secure your core, and maintain an upright position. Be sure your feet remain flat on the floor to ensure your hips and lower body feel stable.
2. Bring your hands to your hips.
3. Slowly push your chest up, and lean back with your upper body.
4. Extend your back until you feel an easy stretch in your upper abdomen and upper back areas.
5. Hold for 10 to 20 seconds.

Release the stretch, and repeat three to five times, or for whatever is most comfortable.

STRETCHING EXERCISES- BEGINNER STRETCHES
SEATED OVERHEAD STRETCH

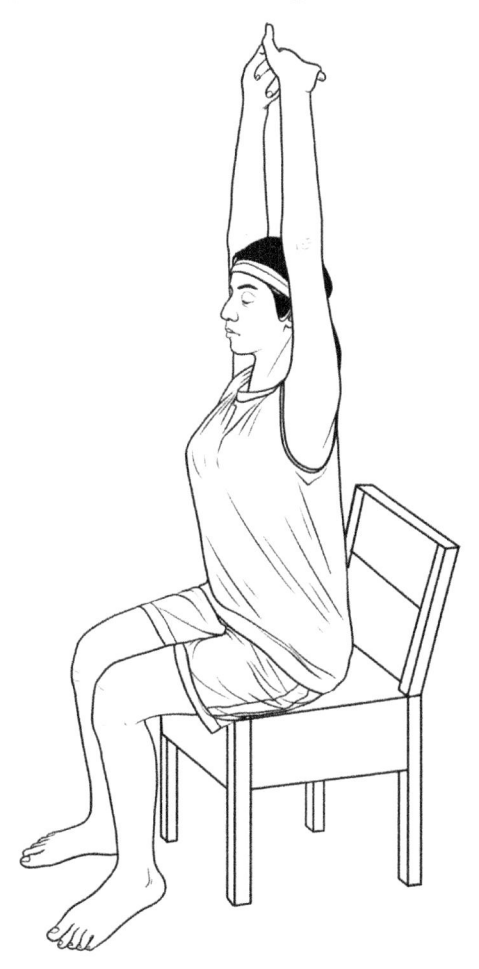

INSTRUCTIONS

1. Sit comfortably in your chair close to the edge. Sit straight to lengthen your spine to secure your core, and maintain an upright position. Keep your feet flat on the floor to ensure your hips and lower body feel stable.
2. Place your hands on your hips to start.
3. Raise both hands from your hips to over your head.
4. Interlock your fingers over your head.
5. Gently arch your back to push your stomach and chest out as you would in a chair yoga cat pose for stretching your abdomen.
6. Hold the stretch for 10 to 20 seconds.

Release the stretch, and repeat three to five times, or for whatever is most comfortable.

STRETCHING EXERCISES- BEGINNER STRETCHES

SEATED HIP STRETCH

INTRODUCTION

Did you know that there are at least 20 different muscles that move through the hip? This includes your abductors, hip flexors, and adductors. In most workout routines, these groups of muscles are often forgotten about, which can lead to injury. When our hips become tight, we lose the ability to bend forward, and our spine can overcompensate. Making sure our hips remain flexible is vital, especially when balancing.

Performing a hip stretch will help if you find it hard to move your legs, waddle while you walk, or have pain in your hip's general area.

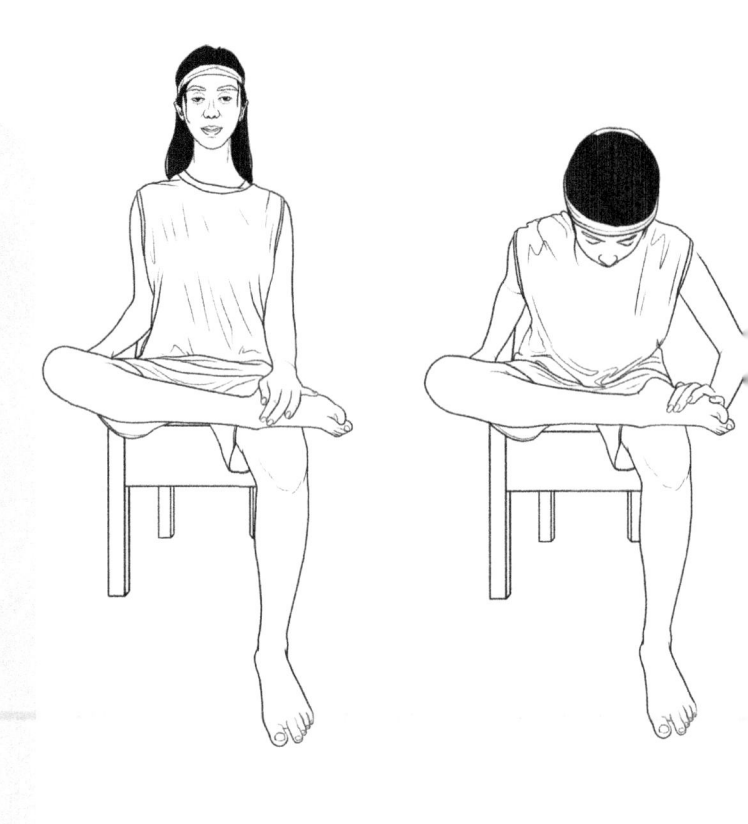

INSTRUCTIONS

1. Sit in your chair with your back upright and your feet flat on the floor. Make sure to engage your core muscles.
2. Cross your right leg over your left to create a triangle between your legs. Your ankle should be just past your left knee.
3. Slowly bend your upper body forward, while maintaining a straight spine and a tight core.
4. Stop when you feel resistance in your glutes or hips. Hold for 10 to 20 seconds before you switch sides.

↻ Repeat three to five times, or whatever feels most comfortable.

STRETCHING EXERCISES- MEDIUM LEVEL STRETCH

SEATED SIDE STRETCH

INTRODUCTION

This stretching exercise is more commonly used in yoga. It helps to stretch out your oblique muscles, neck, back, and shoulders.

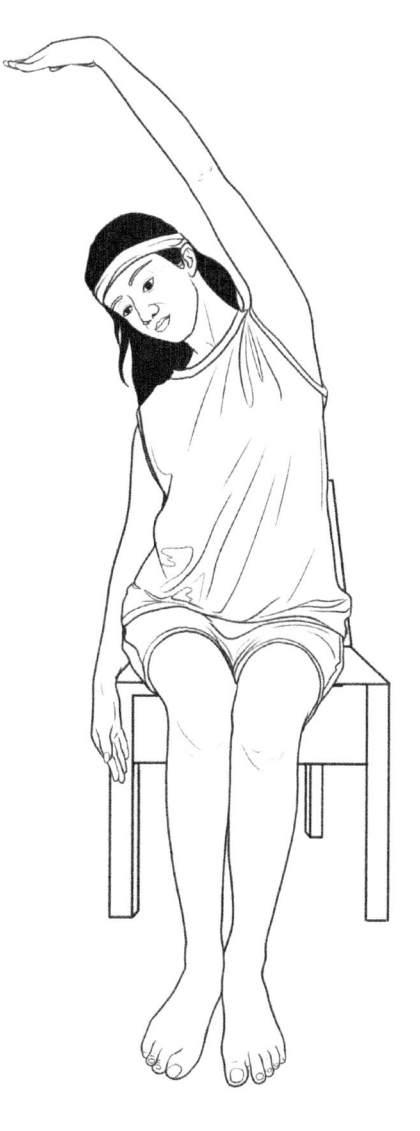

INSTRUCTIONS

1. Sit comfortably in your chair close to the edge. Sit up straight to lengthen your spine to secure your core, and maintain an upright position. Keep your feet flat on the floor to ensure your hips and lower body feel stable.
2. Grip the sides of your chair.
3. Extend the left hand above the head to create a lengthened 'C' shape.
4. Hold the stretch for 10 to 20 seconds.

Release the stretch, and repeat three to five times or whatever is most comfortable.

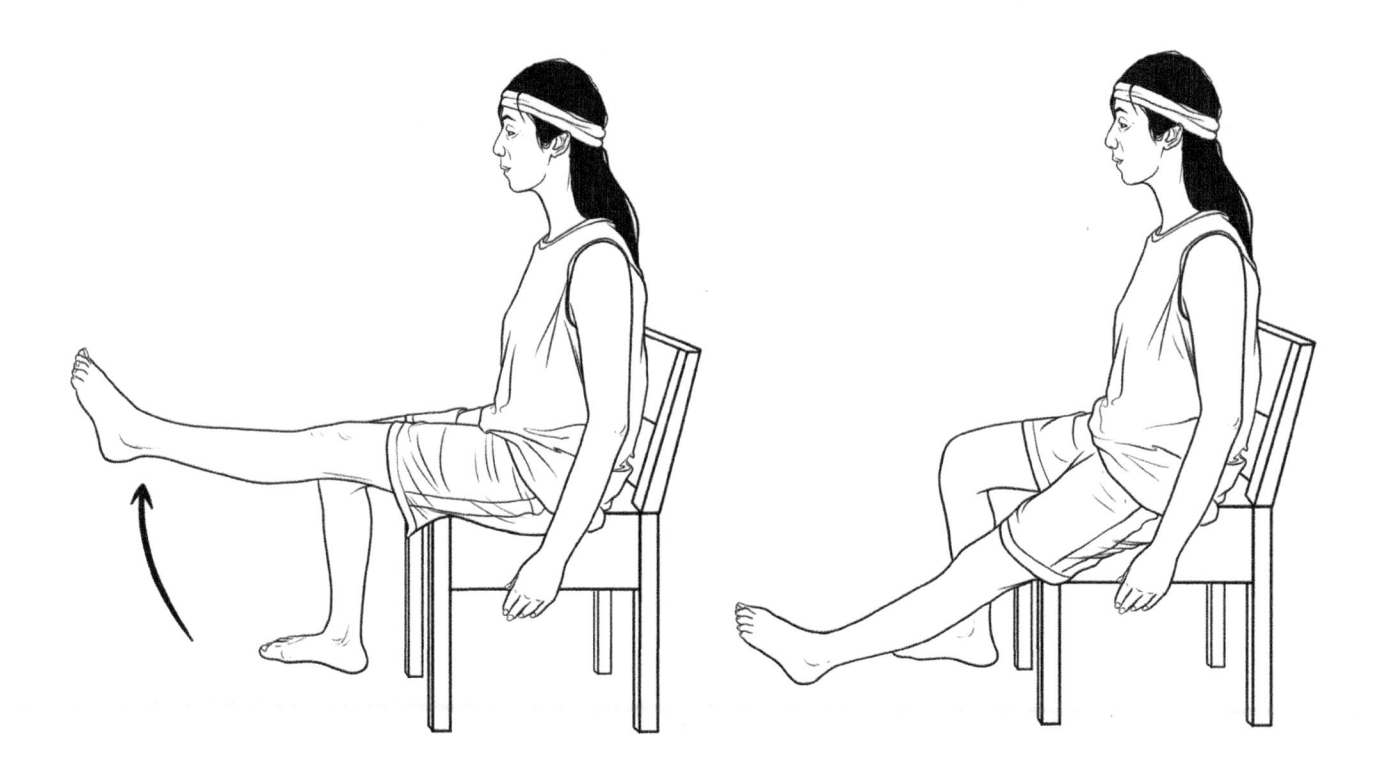

CHAIR EXERCISES- EASY CHAIR EXERCISES
CHAIR LEG RAISES

INTRODUCTION

The chair leg raises will help strengthen your hip flexors and leg muscles.

INSTRUCTIONS

1. Sitting in your chair, lengthen your spine to maintain an upright position.
2. Lift your right leg about five inches off the floor, and hold for five seconds
3. Lower your leg to place your foot back on the floor.
4. Repeat on the left side.

Repeat this for about three to five minutes to activate your hip flexors and leg muscles.

CHAIR EXERCISES- EASY CHAIR EXERCISES

SEATED KNEE-TO-CHEST

INTRODUCTION

The seated knee-to-chest is an excellent exercise to stretch your lower back and lumbar spine muscles. This exercise can also help release any tension in the spinal nerves, and create space for nerves leaving the spine area.

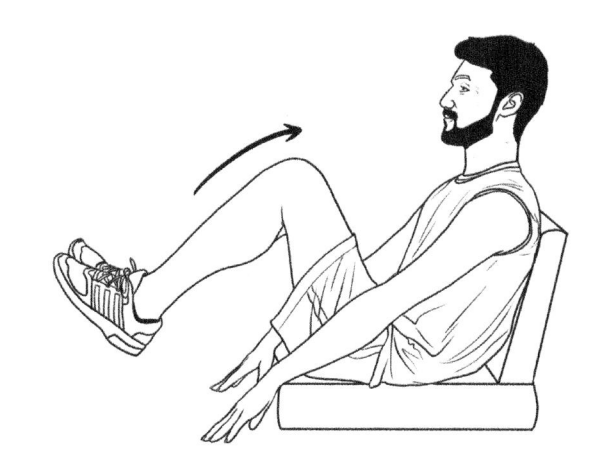

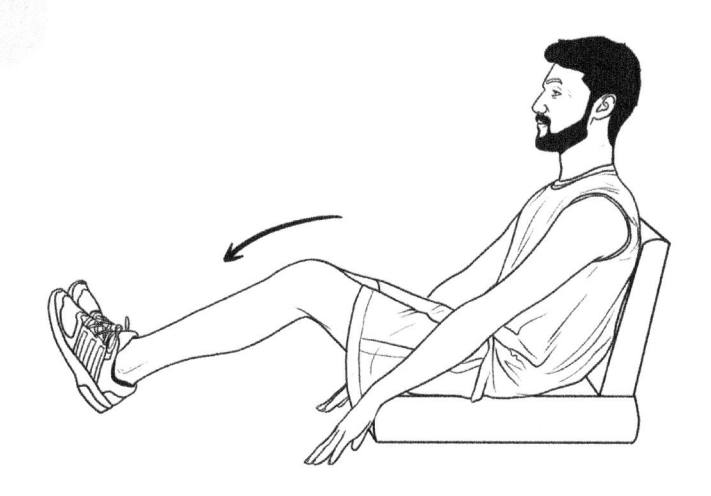

INSTRUCTIONS

1. Sit comfortably on the edge of the chair. You should feel like you are not going to fall forward. Straighten your spine, and engage your core muscles to tighten your lumbar. Stick your chest out, and grip the sides of your seat to remain stable.
2. Extend both legs far out from your body while pointing your toes toward the ceiling. Your legs should be diagonal to your hips.
3. Raise your knees toward your body while bending your knees. Your goal is to have your knees as close to your chest as possible. Remember to listen to your body, and only go as far as is comfortable.
4. Move your legs back down to the starting position.

CHAIR EXERCISES- EASY CHAIR EXERCISES

KNEE EXTENSIONS

INTRODUCTION

The knee extension exercise targets your quadriceps muscles. Working on strengthening your knees and quads will help you walk with ease. This exercise is also excellent if you deal with arthritis in your knee.

INSTRUCTIONS

1. Sit as far back as possible in your chair to ensure your back is against the backrest. Engage your core to keep your lumbar and abdomen muscles tight.
2. With both hands on either side of the seat, stick your chest out. Place your legs at a 90-degree angle.
3. Extend one leg up in front of your body, ensuring that your leg is in line with the hip. Your supporting leg should feel stable as you extend your leg.
4. Slowly bring your leg back down, and repeat on the other side.

Both legs could count as one rep in your sets. In total, you should complete 8-12 sets with each leg.

CHAIR EXERCISES- EASY CHAIR EXERCISES

HEEL SLIDES

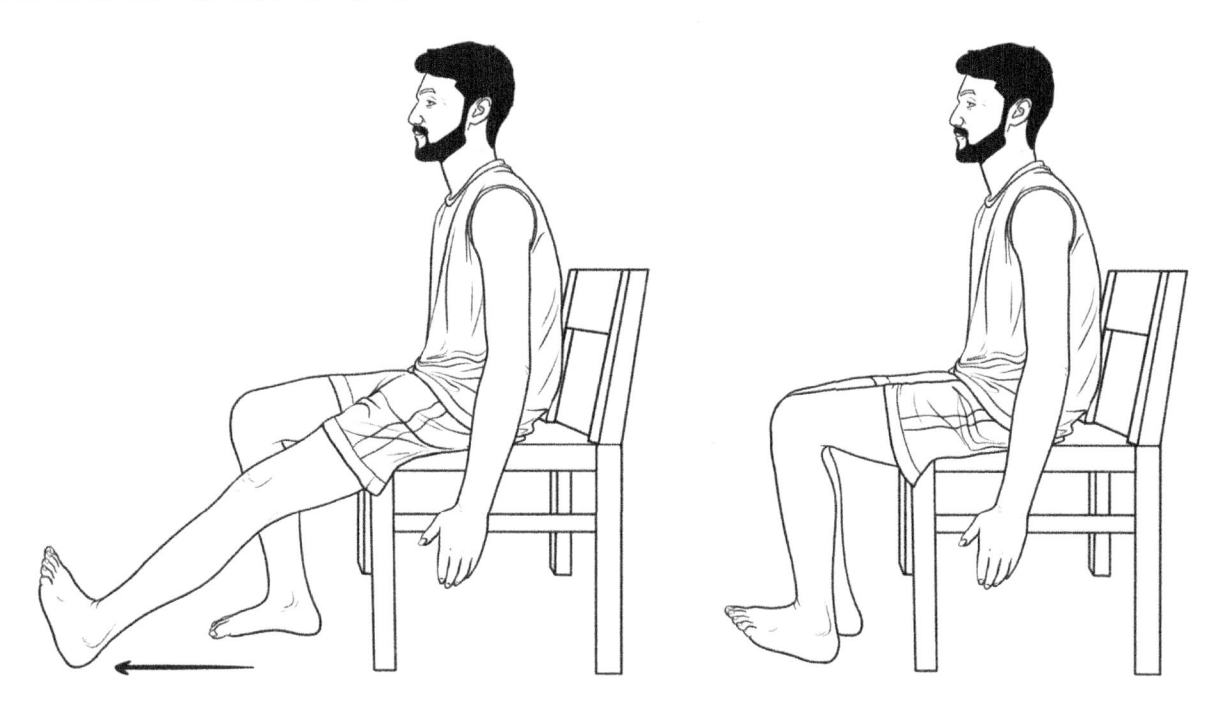

INTRODUCTION

Special note regarding this exercise—if you are having troubles with your knees, it is best to avoid the heel slide exercise, as it could add pressure to your joints.

INSTRUCTIONS

1. Sit comfortably on your chair toward the edge of the seat, making sure you are not so close that you could fall. Engage your core to tighten your abdomen and lumbar. Put your hands on both sides of the seat.
2. Your legs should begin at 90-degrees, your toes pointing forwward.
Slide your foot out until your leg is diagonal to your hips.
3. Drag your foot back to the start. Repeat on the same leg.

↻ The repetitions in this exercise equate to one forward and backward motion with your leg. Move your first leg 8-12 times before switching to the other to complete one set.

CHAIR EXERCISES- EASY CHAIR EXERCISES

SEATED CALF RAISES

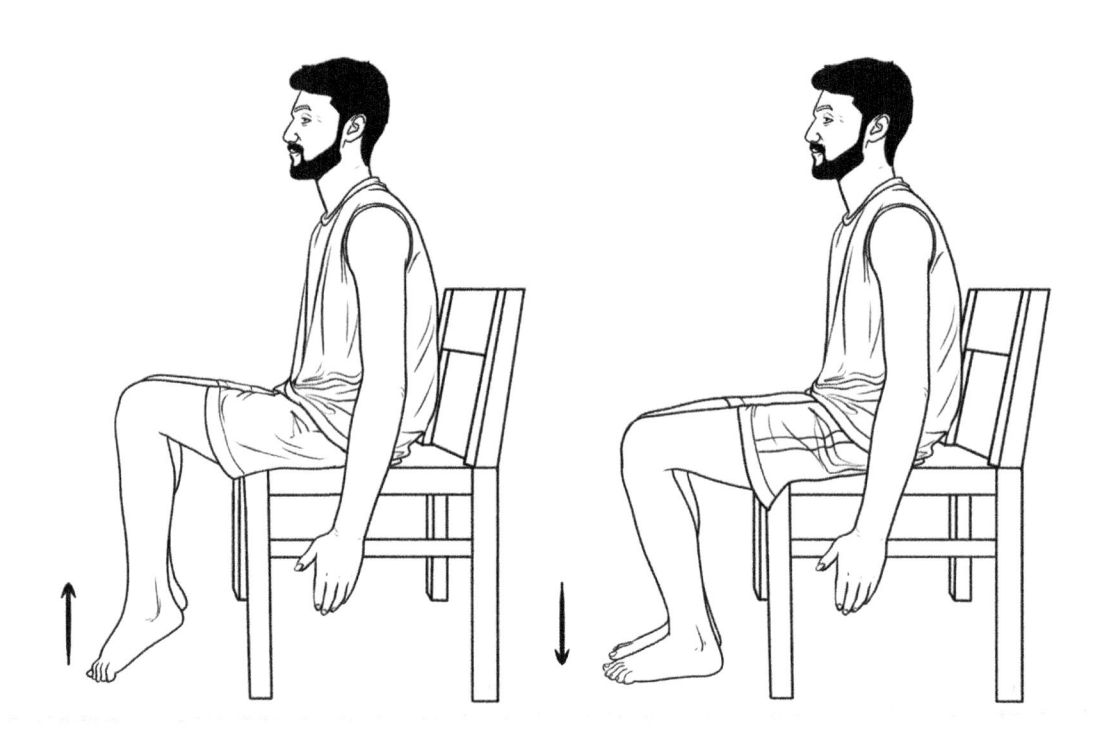

INTRODUCTION

Doing calf raises from a seated position is a great stretch to help your tight joints and muscles around your lower leg.

INSTRUCTIONS

1. In your chair, sit as far back as you can with your back against the backrest.
2. Engage your core muscles to provide stability around your abdomen and lumbar. Stick your chest out, and place your hands on either side, just as you have done in the previous exercises.
3. Your legs should be bent at 90 degrees, with your feet flat on your floor.
4. Extend the heels of your feet upward by pushing your toes on the floor.
5. Lower your heels to the floor, then repeat.

You will do this exercise three times, with 20 repetitions in each set.

CHAIR EXERCISES- MEDIUM TO ADVANCED CHAIR EXERCISES

SEATED EXTENDED LEG RAISES

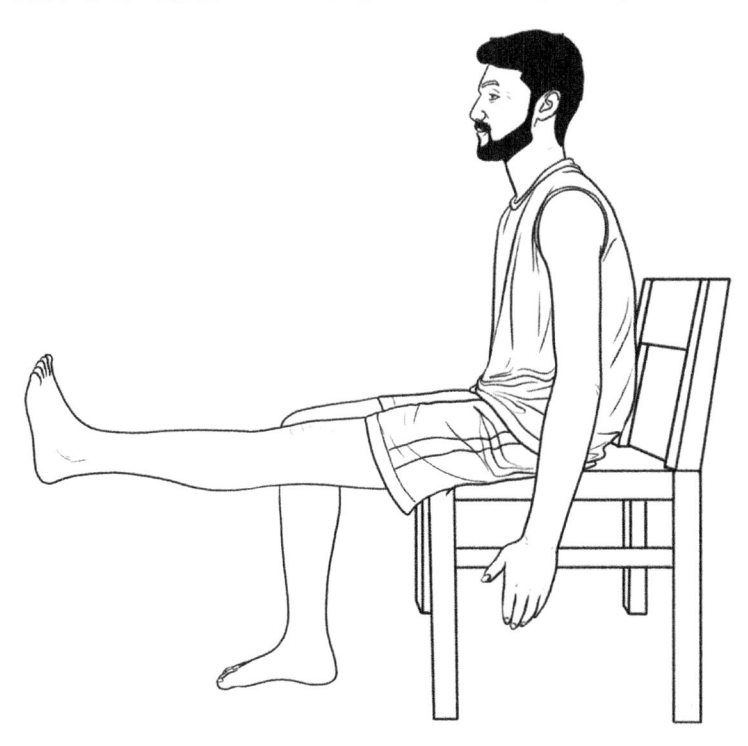

INTRODUCTION

Leg raises help to increase your blood flow, and strengthen and improve your leg and core muscles.

INSTRUCTIONS

1. Sit comfortably on the edge of the chair. Straighten your spine, and engage your core muscles to tighten your lumbar. Stick your chest out, and grip the sides of your seat to remain stable.
2. Extend both your feet in front of the body, with your toes pointed to the ceiling, and heels on the floor. Your legs should be diagonal to your hips.
3. Lift your right leg as high as it is comfortable. The ideal range would be your leg in line with your hip. As you move your leg up, remain centered, and do not move your body. Your left leg is to stay in the starting position.
4. Lower your leg back to the starting position. Repeat the exercise with your left leg going up.

↻ Extending both legs counts as one repetition.

CHAIR EXERCISES- EASY CHAIR EXERCISES

LEG KICKS

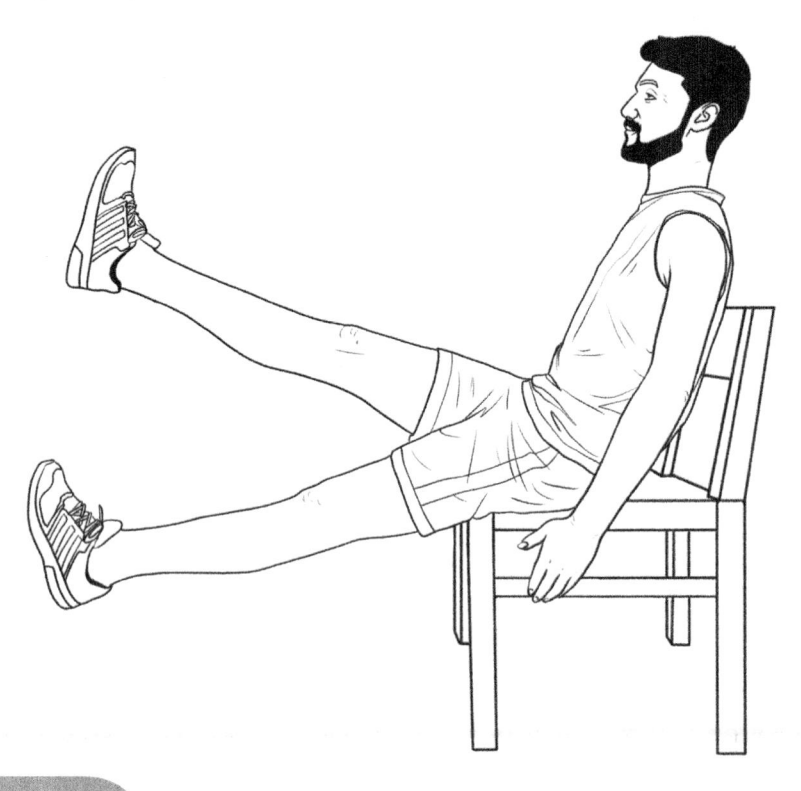

INTRODUCTION

This exercise is similar to the extended leg raises in the movement with an added challenge. Picture yourself swimming in a pool, and kicking your legs in the water.

INSTRUCTIONS

1. Begin by sitting on your chair near the edge. Engage your core muscles to tighten your lumbar and lengthen your spine. Stick your chest out and grip the sides of your seat to remain stable and centered.
2. Extended both legs up and out from your body with toes facing forward in a diagonal.
3. Lean your upper body backward to stabilize your hips.
4. Lift your leg to the highest point that is comfortable. The goal for the exercise would be to have your working leg parallel to your hip.
5. Slowly lower your leg to the floor, and switch to your other leg.

VARIATIONS OF SEATED EXERCISES
SEATED KNEE-TO-CHEST VARIATION

INTRODUCTION

If you find the seated knee-to-chest variation challenging, try isolating the exercise to one leg. Keep one leg planted on the ground before lifting your other knee toward your chest.

VARIATIONS OF SEATED EXERCISES
SEATED EXTENDED LEG RAISES

INTRODUCTION

For a variation on the extended leg raises, try isolating your legs by lifting one at a time, while your supporting leg remains planted on the floor.

CHAPTER FIVE
STANDING EXERCISES

Seated exercises allowed you to avoid using momentum, or the incorrect muscle groups, while you learned the correct technique and form to perform a particular exercise. By sitting, you have the opportunity to cater to an injury, or isolate specific muscle groups as well. On the other hand, stand-up exercises allow you to target specific muscle groups in conjunction with your lower body and core muscles. When you stand, it challenges you to focus on your stability and balance by forcing your core muscles to work harder, while contradicting the weight of the exercise.

Depending on the exercise you are trying, you might want to try using a wall or a chair for support where necessary. However, the exercise instructions will let you know when you might need the support.

TEN EXERCISES THAT YOU CAN DO WHILE STANDING

EASY STANDING EXERCISES
CALF STRETCH

INTRODUCTION

For this exercise you can either use a table, chair, or a wall. If you are going to use a chair, make sure to place the front legs against a wall or have it tucked under your table for stability.

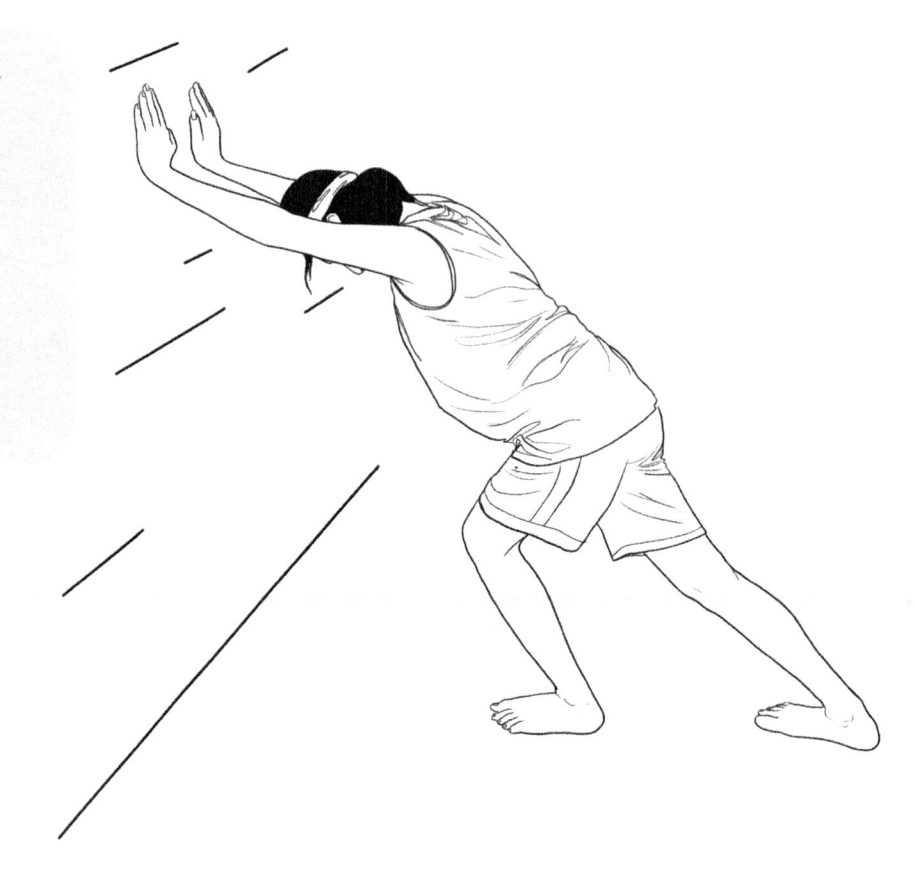

INSTRUCTIONS

1. Holding onto the chair, table, or wall, stand in a lunge position with your front leg bent slightly.
2. Shift your weight forward onto your front supporting leg while you press your back heel into the floor.
3. Hold for 20 seconds and then change to your opposite leg, repeating the same steps.

Helpful tip: move your weight forward more if you need a deeper stretch in your calf. However, be sure to listen to your body if the stretch feels too deep and is causing pain.

EASY STANDING EXERCISES
LADDER

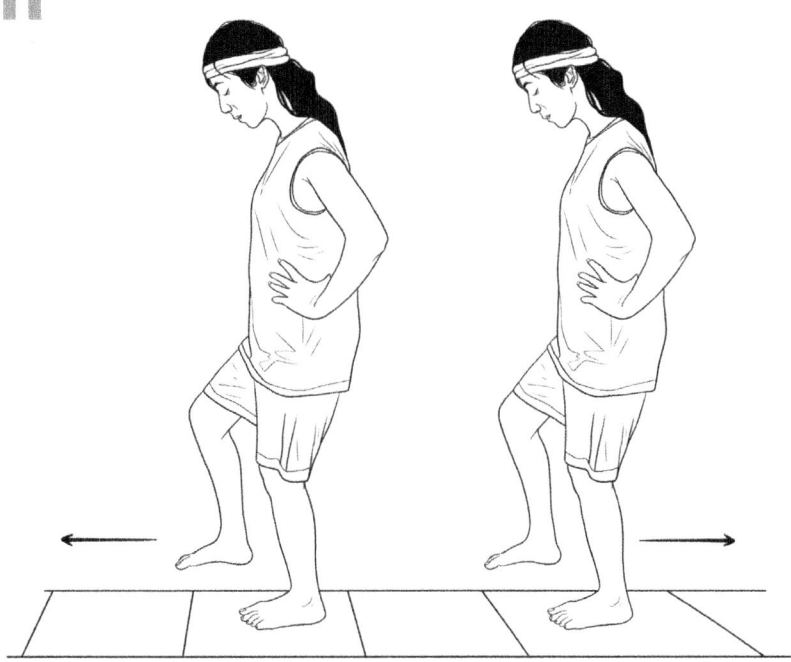

INTRODUCTION

For the ladder exercise, you can use an agility ladder. However, if you don't have an agility ladder, here are some other options you can do to try out this exercise:

Try drawing a ladder outside with sidewalk chalk

Going to the local playground or schoolground where a hopscotch might be on the ground already

Or, imagine you have a ladder in your home

To begin this exercise, start at the base of your agility ladder or the hopscotch.

INSTRUCTIONS

1. Step into the first space of the ladder with your right leg, and then your left.
2. Step back the same way.
3. Continue this motion, adding a rung to each step until you are at the end.

Helpful tip: if you are drawing or imagining the ladder, agility ladders typically have 10 rungs.

EASY STANDING EXERCISES
TOE LIFTS

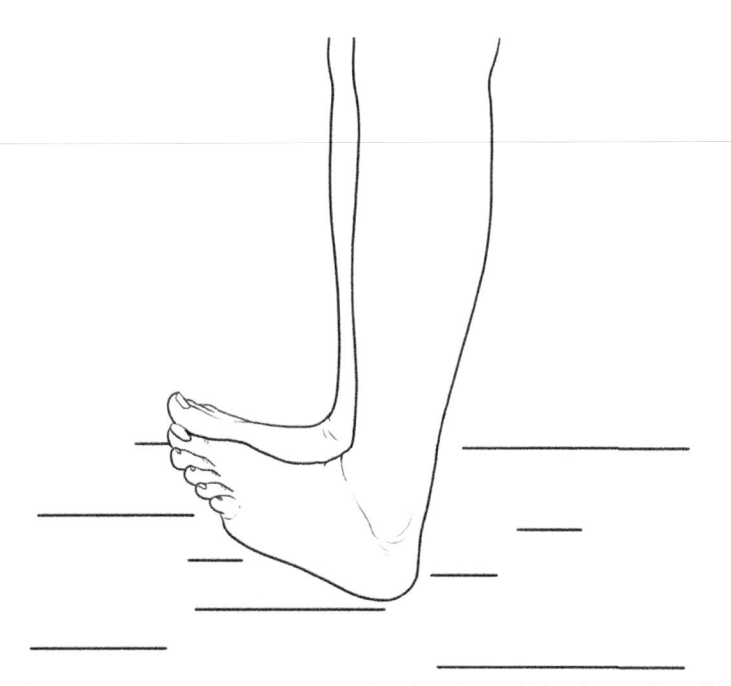

INTRODUCTION

Toe lifts are a great standing exercise to strengthen your lower leg muscles and calves. For this one, you can either use the back of a chair, a wall, or a table or countertop for support.

INSTRUCTIONS

1. Begin by standing behind the chair, place both hands on the backrest.
2. As you would have done in the seated calf raises, lift your heels off the floor to stand on your toes.
3. Hold for 10 seconds before lowering to the floor.

⟳ Repeat 10 times.

EASY STANDING EXERCISES

MARCHING ON THE SPOT

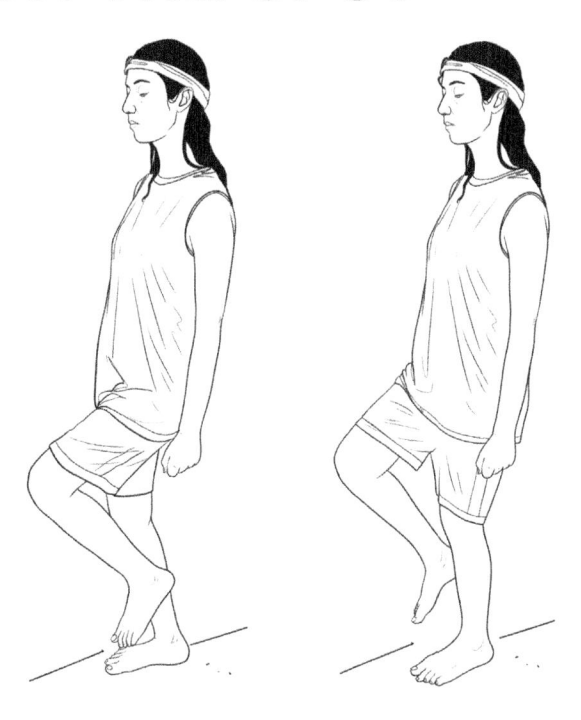

INTRODUCTION

The next time you are watching television or making dinner, try marching on the spot! Not only will this exercise help improve your body awareness when it comes to balancing, you'll also get a light aerobic movement from it. The excellent part about this exercise is that it is one of the more versatile exercises you can do at any point, and easily adaptable when you just want to get a few minutes of exercise in. To make it more fun, play music or see how long you can march in between commercial breaks.

INSTRUCTIONS

1. Lift your right knee to hip level while swinging your left arm out in front of you.
2. Repeat on the other side.
3. Speed the movements up until you are marching on the spot.

↻ As you are marching, make sure to move at a pace that is comfortable to you for one minute, the length of the commercial break, or the whole song.

MEDIUM STANDING EXERCISES
ROCK THE BOAT

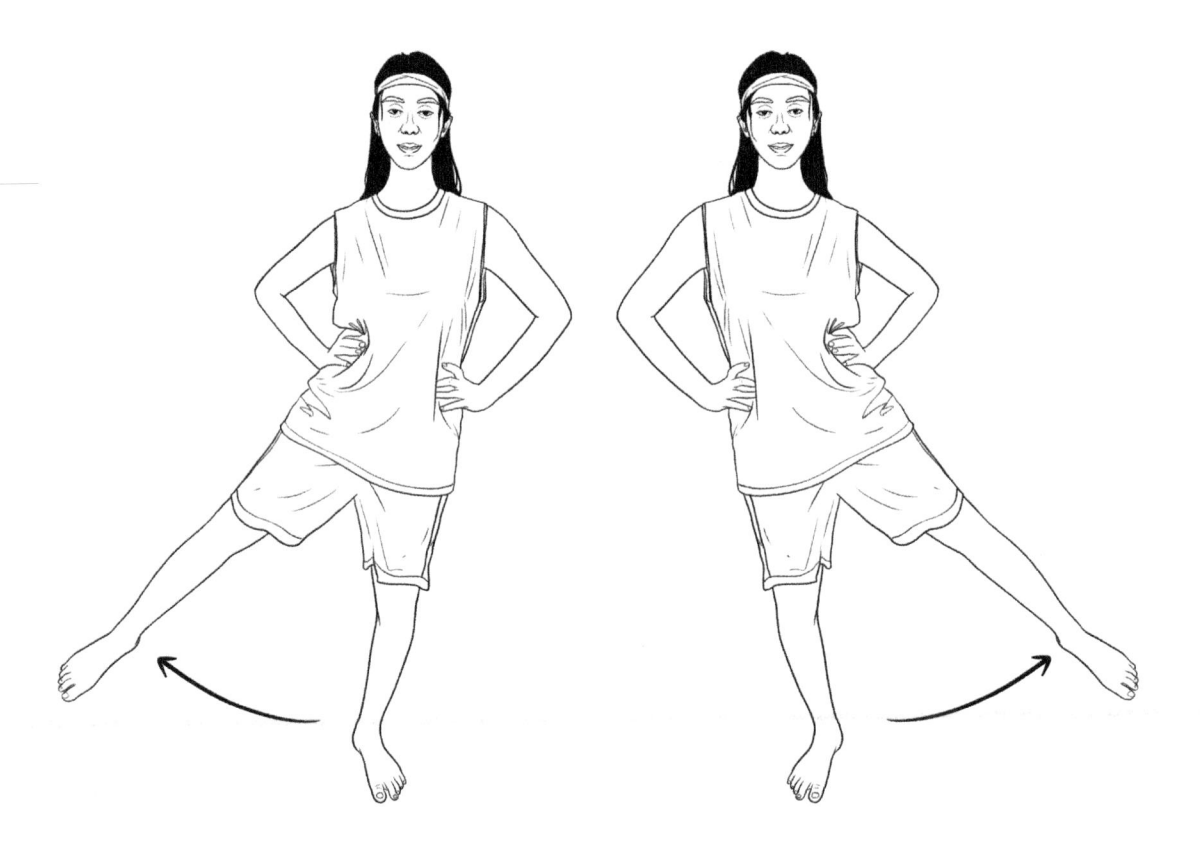

INTRODUCTION

Rock the boat helps to address your balancing issues by standing on one leg, and leaning in the opposite direction. For this exercise, you will need a chair for support.

INSTRUCTIONS

1. Face the back of your chair. Put your hands on the chair's backrest.
2. Lift your right leg to the side and lean towards the left. There should be a diagonal line from the top of your head down to your heel.
3. Hold for five seconds before returning to center.
4. Repeat with your left leg.

For this exercise, do each leg 10 times in two to three sets.

MEDIUM STANDING EXERCISES
SIDE-STEP WALK

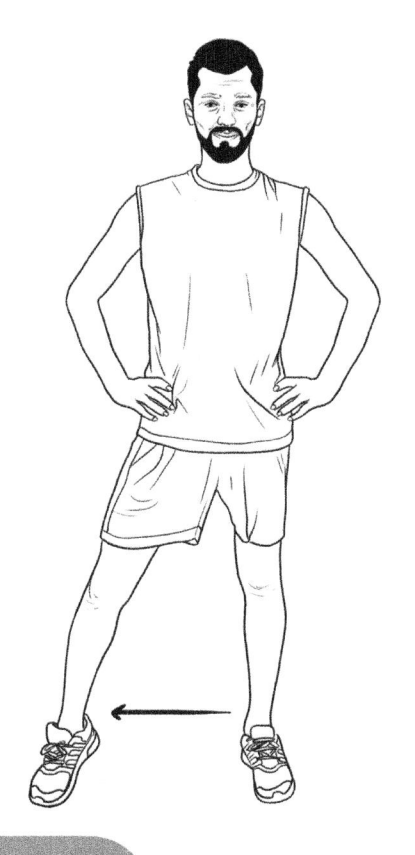

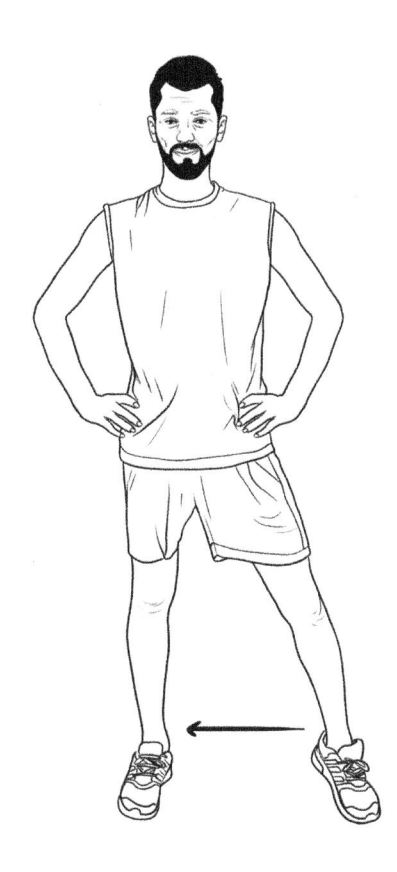

INTRODUCTION

Taking steps to the side not only challenges your balance in a lateral movement, but it also can help improve the stability of your feet, ankle, knee and hips.

INSTRUCTIONS

1. Standing in the center of the room, step out sideways with your right leg, bringing your left foot to meet it.
2. Step back to the center with your left leg, bringing your right leg to meet it.
3. Repeat to your left, repeating the same pattern.

Try doing 15 to 20 steps total in each direction. For an added challenge, try moving laterally across the room and then moving back in the opposite direction.

MEDIUM STANDING EXERCISES
STEPPING STONES

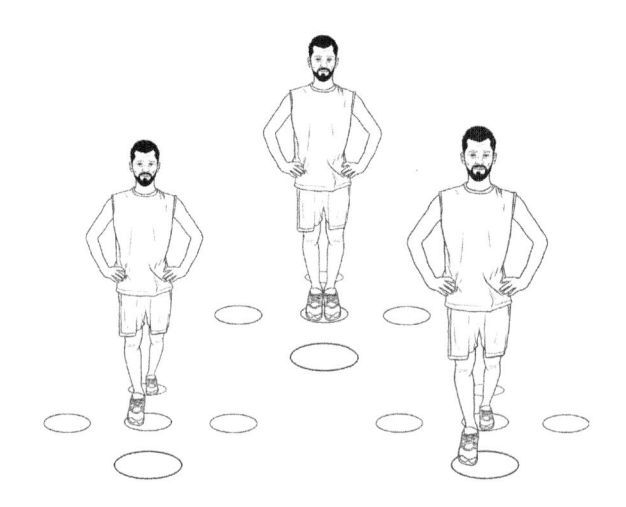

INTRODUCTION

The stepping stones exercise has you practice stepping over objects. For the stepping stones exercise, you will need five circle markers (like hula hoops or circles drawn on the floor) to be placed around you. They need to be big enough for you to step into. You might want to use a cane if necessary.

To set up this exercise, start with one circle in the middle. Next, you will put one circle in front, one at the back, and one at either side. Picture it as if you were to turn a die with the five sides up on an angle.

INSTRUCTIONS

1. Start in the center circle.
2. Use your right leg to step into the circle behind you. Bring your left foot backward to complete the step.
3. Step forward into the starting circle with your right leg and then your left.
4. Next, step to the right circle marker with your left leg to finish.
5. Go back to the center.
6. Step to your left following the same pattern.
7. Return to the center hoop.

↻ Repeat this exercise for three minutes.

MEDIUM STANDING EXERCISES
STEP UPS

INTRODUCTION

The step up exercise can even out imbalances in your body as it is a unilateral leg exercise. In this movement, you will step up on a step one leg at a time to target your body evenly. What you will find is that your attention will be brought to any muscle imbalances you have between your two sides. The exercise will also help with your stability when you work on engaging your core and lower back muscles during the movement. For the step ups exercise, you will need a low step stool (placed against the wall), or you can use the bottom step of a staircase. You are encouraged to use a cane or the back of a chair for support as you step up and down. Here is how to do this simple and effective exercise!

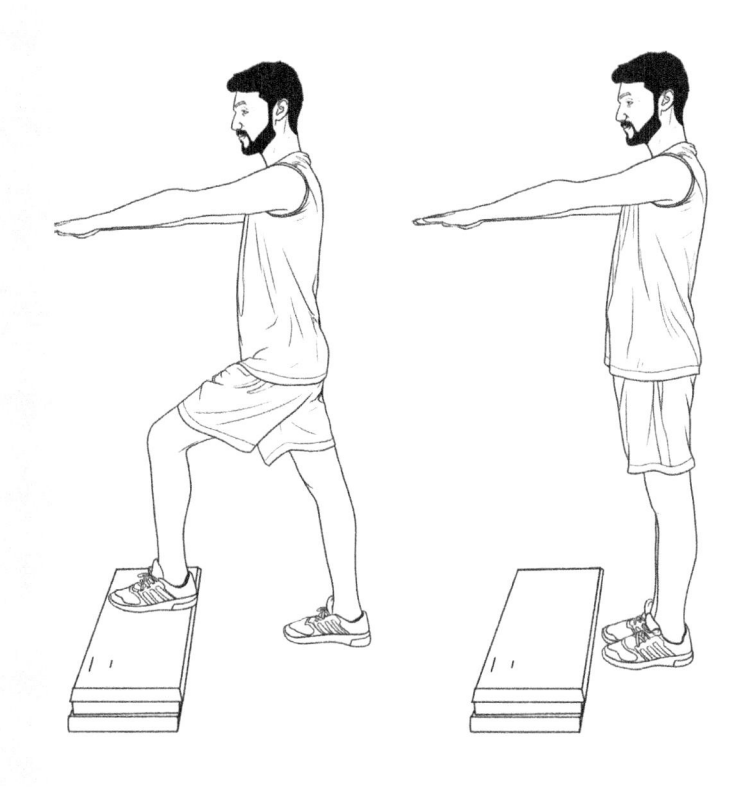

INSTRUCTIONS

1. Standing in front of your step, step up using your right leg, and then bring your left up to match it.
2. Step down in the same order.

Repeat this exercise 15 to 20 times.

MEDIUM STANDING EXERCISES

STANDING BACK LEG RAISES

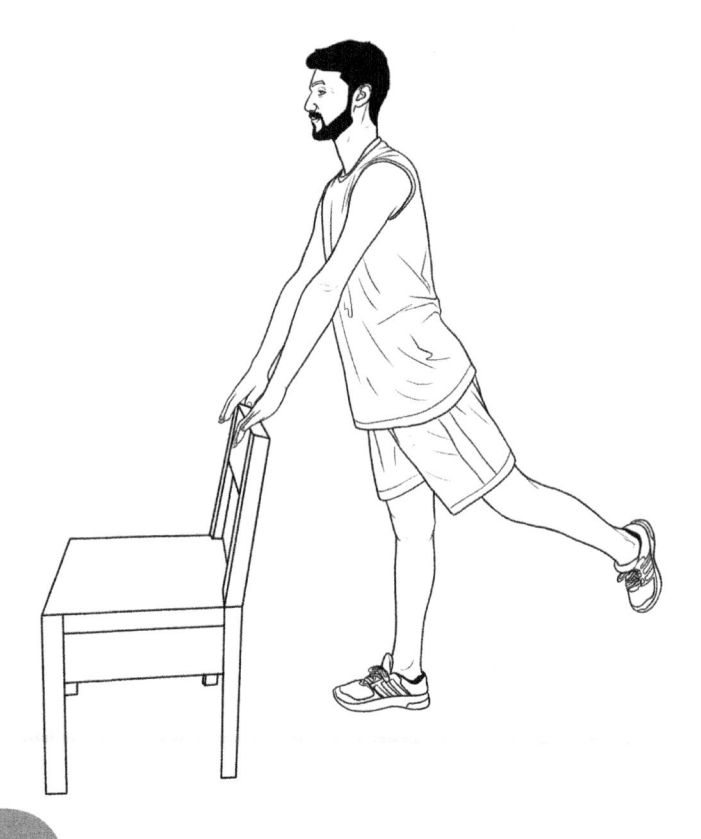

INTRODUCTION

Back leg raises have an array of benefits to improving your overall balance. The exercise is done standing on one leg, with your working leg moving to the back. In addition, you will find that the back leg raises help strengthen your glutes, and your lower back muscles. For this exercise, use the back of a chair for support.

INSTRUCTIONS

1. Shift your weight to your left leg.
2. Lift your right leg about two inches off of the floor behind you, keeping your ankle loose.
3. Hold for 10 seconds before lowering back to the floor.
4. Repeat on other side.

↻ For this exercise, lift each leg 10-15 times in two to three sets.

MEDIUM STANDING EXERCISES
SIDE LEG RAISES

INTRODUCTION

Side leg raises will help target your hip flexors and thighs while challenging your core to keep you upright. In addition, the movement will help with your flexibility. In this exercise, you are encouraged to use the back of your chair, wall, or countertop for support.

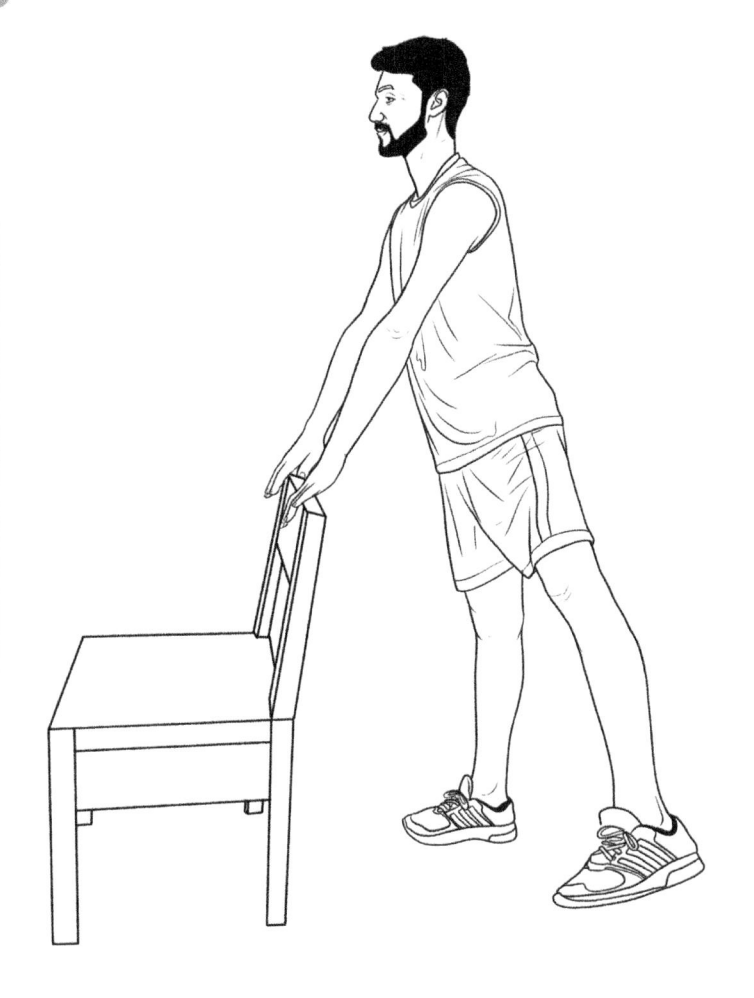

INSTRUCTIONS

1. Stand facing the back of your chair.
2. Elevate your right leg out to the side and hold for 10 seconds.
3. Lower and repeat with your left leg.

↻ Repeat with lifting each leg 10-15 times for two to three sets.

CHAPTER SIX

WALKING EXERCISES

Some people can find walking boring, especially if you are walking the same route where you live. However, there are many ways to make your walks enjoyable, such as walking in nature. For example, when you walk along a creek, river, beach, or hiking trail in a forest, you will not only get a change of scenery, but your body will be challenged on different terrain. Outside walking also contributes to improving your mental health, as well as giving you some fresh air.

If you cannot get to a beach or outside, try a different challenge on your route! Bring some light weights, increase your pace, or use the elevation to your advantage!

In addition, here are some other benefits walking has for you:

- Walking can help improve your overall heart health. When you walk, either leisurely or on a brisk 15 to 20-minute walk, you can help maintain a healthy weight, invigorate your metabolism, and lower your blood cholesterol, all of which contribute to a healthy heart and reduce your risk of heart disease

- Your stress will be lowered when you walk more frequently! It is no secret that we face some stressful moments in our week, and many factors contribute to feeling stressed. When stress happens, our bodies create cortisol, suppressing our immune system. However, a neat chemical called endorphins is released when you go for a walk! Endorphins work with the brain's receptors to bring out good feelings surrounding your well-being and self-esteem

- When we walk (and work out regularly), it is believed that the change in the antibodies in our systems and our white blood cells are factors in fighting off common illnesses such as a cold or a flu. In any exercise, especially walking, our body temperature will also temporarily rise. With the change in temperature, bacteria, especially in our gut, are less likely to grow, slowing down the stress hormone cortisol

- The strength of your joints can also be improved through walking while helping or treating osteoarthritis. Walking can also help with your pain tolerance, because you move your joints with each step

- Your blood sugar will be better controlled. One meta-analysis tested 300,000 participants and found that 30% had a lower risk of developing Type 2 diabetes when walking regularly. Of those participants living with the disease, adding 2,600 steps per day helped lower their blood sugar levels by 0.2%

If you want to increase your walking, try taking the stairs instead of the elevator or escalator. Remember, when walking on the stairs, you focus on your balance between each side of your body. You can also park far away from the mall or store entrance while running errands.

TEN EXERCISES THAT YOU CAN DO WHILE WALKING

Not every day is going to be the perfect weather to go outside. Here are 10 exercises that can help you get your steps in!

EASY WALKING EXERCISES

MARCHING ON THE SPOT WITH ARMS

INTRODUCTION

In chapter five, you marched on the spot as you might see a navy march. This version, however, includes a stretch both upwards and sideways to lengthen your spine and open your chest, and therefore is a slow-motion version. Your arms going upwards and sideways will still challenge your balancing technique.

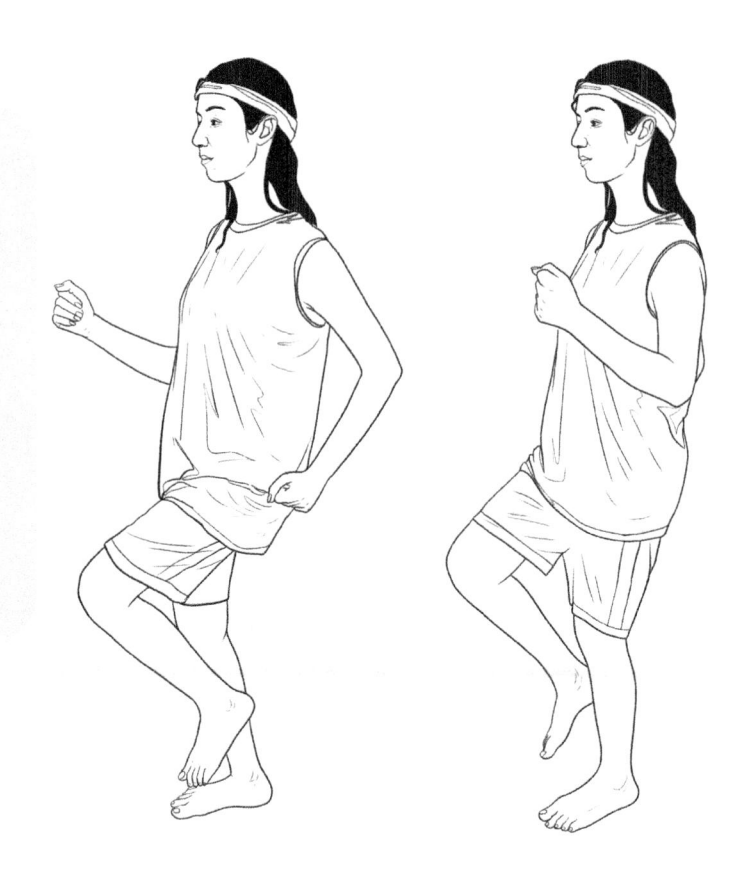

INSTRUCTIONS

For the upwards motion:
1. Lift your right knee to hip level, while lifting both arms into the air.
2. Lower your leg and switch to the other side, repeating the same motion.

For the sideways motion of your arms, repeat the same steps, except that you will open your arms wide in a 'T' shape and then cross them as if you are hugging yourself. As you lift your other leg, you will re-open them wide. If you cannot raise your leg to hip height, don't worry about it. Always listen to your body, and lift your leg to what is most comfortable.

EASY WALKING EXERCISES

SIDE-TO-SIDE TAPS

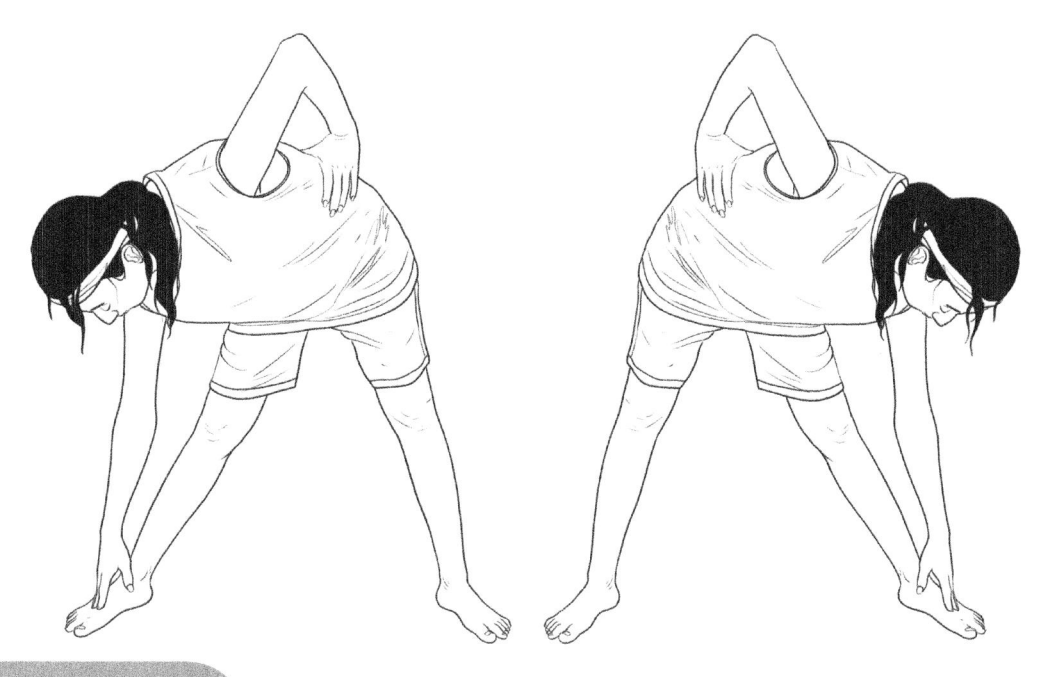

INTRODUCTION

This exercise is a level up from the side-to-side walks you tried in Chapter five, with a little more fun to the steps, and a slightly elevated heart rate. You will need enough space for this exercise as you step your leg from side to side.

INSTRUCTIONS

1. Starting in the middle of your room or space, step your right foot out, and tap your toes on the floor. Your foot should be facing the front.
2. Bring your right foot in.
3. Step your left foot out, making the same motion.

Complete the same pattern for one minute. Alternatively, you can play some music, and sidestep to the beat. For an added challenge, add some arms. Bending them at 90 degrees, bring them up to shoulder height, and lower down as you bring your foot in. Next, lift your bent arms to shoulder height as you tap your opposite foot.

EASY WALKING EXERCISES
LATERAL STEP

INTRODUCTION

The lateral step is a little similar to the side-to-side walk, except this time with a more aerobic flair and movement. Again, make sure you have space to move. For some extra fun, try using music to keep a beat.

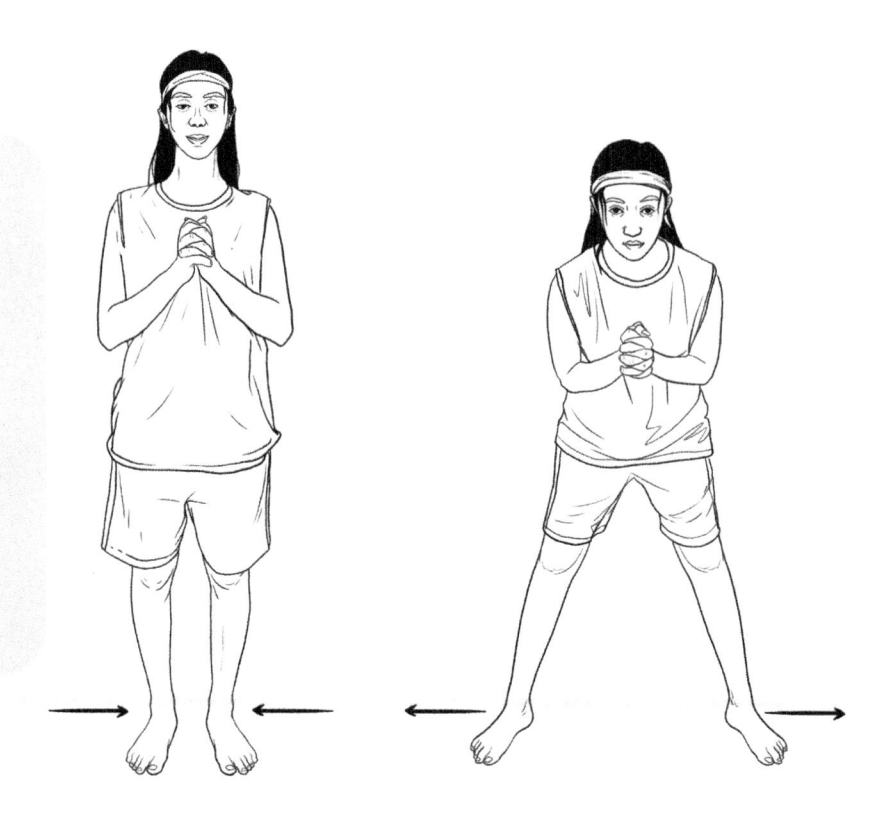

INSTRUCTIONS

1. Step out with your right foot in the middle of your room or space.
2. Next, step out with your left foot, so your stance is slightly wider than your hips. Remember to listen to your body, and avoid going wider than your body likes.
3. Step in with your right, then step in with your left.

↻ Repeat for a minute, or the duration of the song. You may keep your hands by your sides or at 90 degrees, to pump as you take a step (as you might do in a brisk walk). If you have some balance issues, try using a cane for support.

EASY WALKING EXERCISES
HEEL TOUCHES

INTRODUCTION

Heel touches are an excellent activity to focus on balancing both sides of your body, while activating your upper and lower abdomen muscles. It's fun to do too, especially to music. For the heel touches exercise, you want some space, but you don't need a lot of it. You could also try this exercise during commercial breaks, or while cooking dinner!

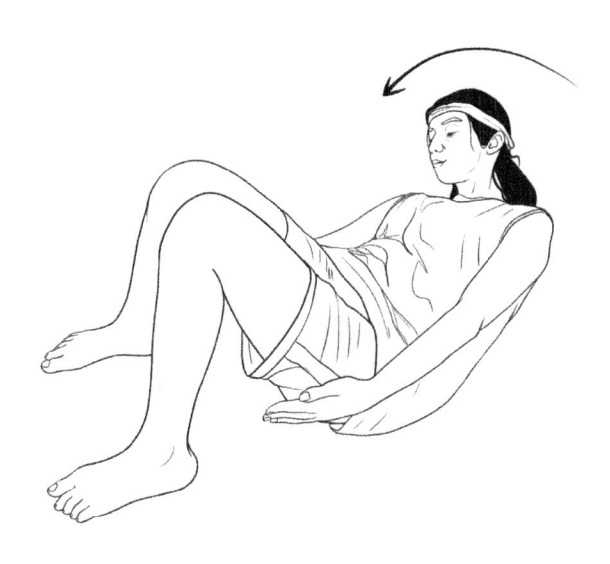

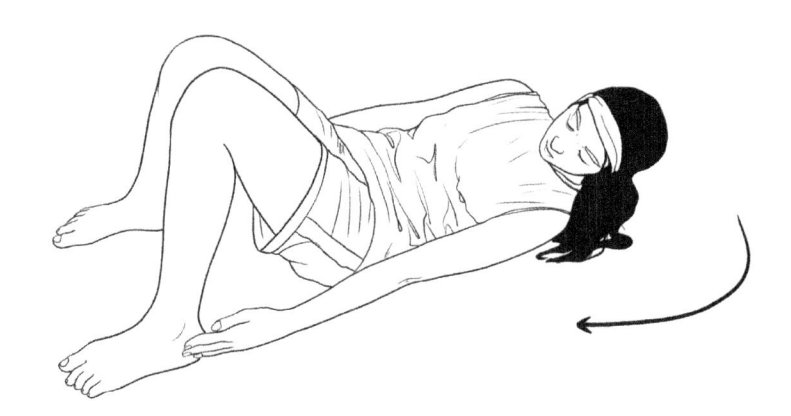

INSTRUCTIONS

1. In the middle of the room or space, bring your right foot forward, and touch your heel to the ground with your toes facing the ceiling.
2. Bring your right foot back, and repeat with your left foot.

Repeat this exercise for a minute, or challenge yourself to go for the whole song if you decide to do it to music. Again, your hands can remain neutral at your sides, or you may wish to bring them to 90 degrees as done in the lateral steps.

EASY WALKING EXERCISES

HEEL-TO-TOE TOUCHES

INTRODUCTION

The heel-to-toe touches challenge your balance, and this exercise will also challenge you mentally! You will want enough space to walk forwards and backward. Using a table, countertop, or cane is recommended for stability.

INSTRUCTIONS

1. Begin to walk forward with your right leg for three steps.
2. On the fourth step, tap your left heel out front with your toes toward the ceiling. Step back with your left leg for three steps.
3. On the fourth, tap the ball of your foot to the floor.
4. Repeat for one minute, then switch sides, with your left foot leading you forward and right foot leading you backward.

↻ Do this exercise for at least a minute. You are encouraged to go longer if you feel like it!

MEDIUM WALKING EXERCISES
KNEE UPS

INTRODUCTION

Knee ups are a modified version of high knees. The exercise will help improve your cardio through a light aerobic workout, and boost your lower body's endurance and overall coordination! Just make sure to have enough room to move.

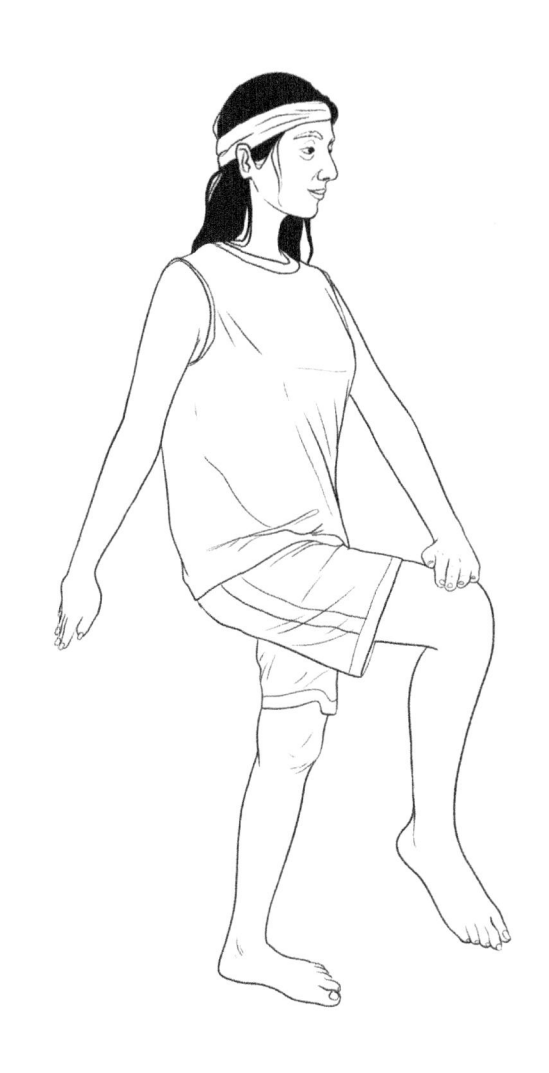

INSTRUCTIONS

1. Bend your knee and bring your right leg up while simultaneously bringing your left hand to meet it.
2. Lower your arm and leg to switch sides.

↻ If you can, try to have your knee aligned with your hip. If this is not possible, don't worry about it! You can keep your arms at the side, while you lift your leg as high as is comfortable for you. If you feel your balance is off, use a chair for support.

MEDIUM WALKING EXERCISES
ZIG-ZAG WALKING

INTRODUCTION

Walking in a zig-zag pattern will challenge you mentally as you shift from one direction to the next. In addition, the exercise will help strengthen the muscles in your lower legs. You might find this exercise similar to the heel-to-toe walking from Chapter three. In this exercise, you'll need enough space to take five steps in one direction before switching to another. It is probably best to do this one outside!

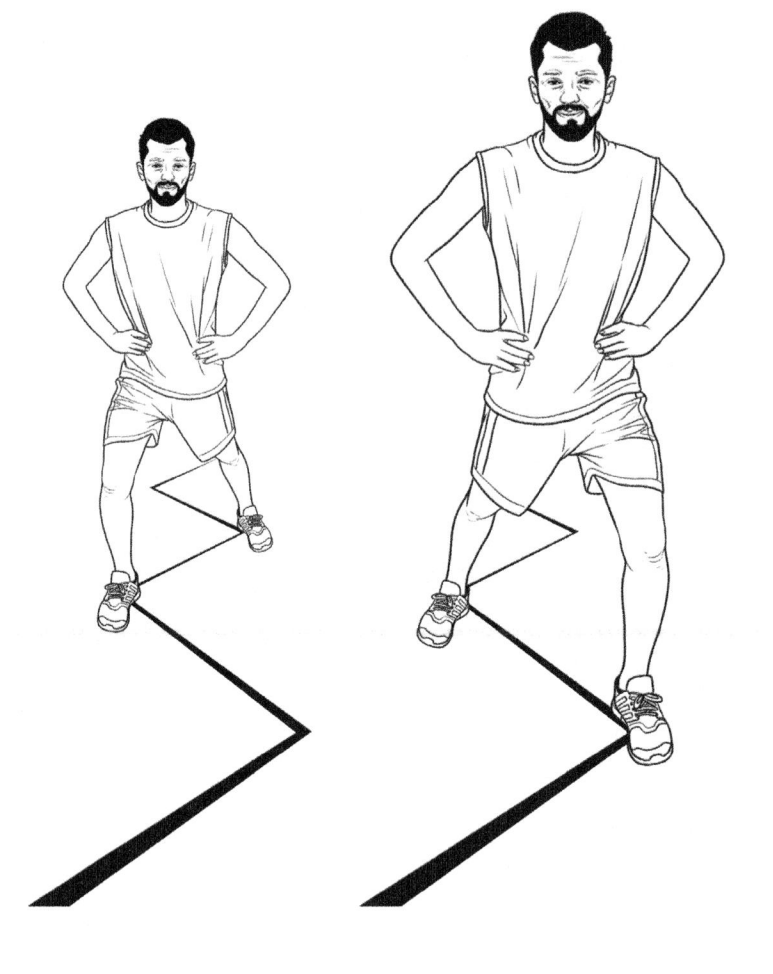

INSTRUCTIONS

1. Stand up straight on one side of the room, or the side you will begin on if you are outside.
2. Begin walking to the left by crossing your right leg in front of the left leg, to walk in one direction.
3. Continue to cross your legs in front of one another, to touch your heel to your toe for five steps; then change direction and take another five steps.

↻ Each time you change direction, your feet should alternate to lead you. For example, when you change direction with your left foot, you should go to your right.

MEDIUM WALKING EXERCISES
OBSTACLES

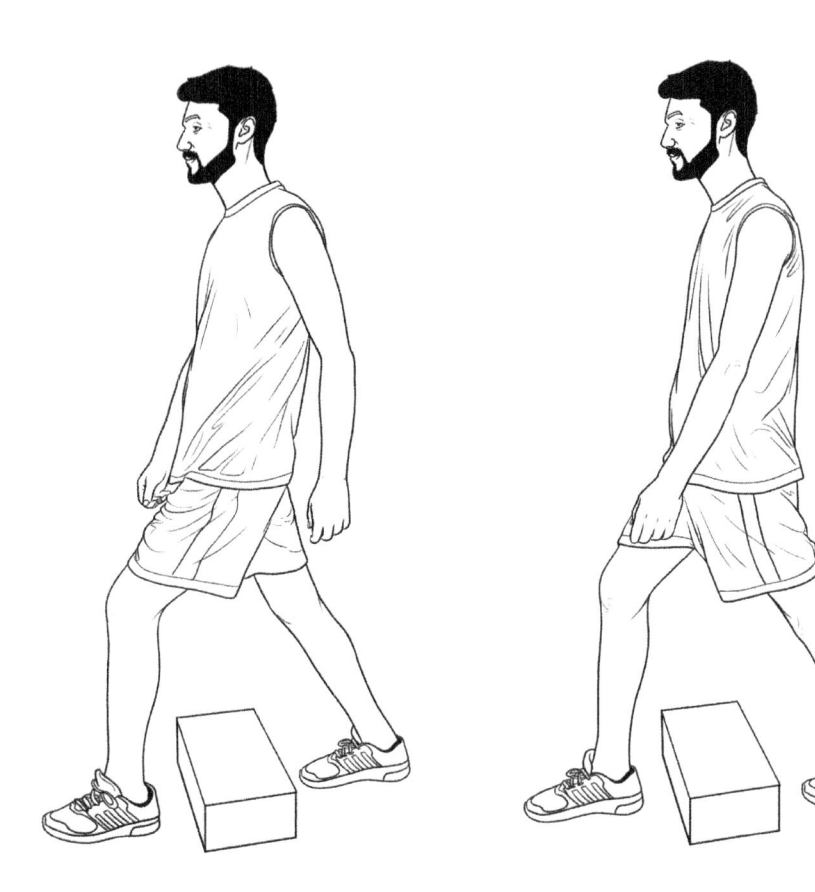

INTRODUCTION

The obstacle exercise is an opportunity to practice stepping over objects, which seniors sometimes have difficulty with, resulting in a fall. You can grab anything for this exercise to place in front of you, such as a small pillow, a grandchild's stuffed animal, or maybe a dog's bone. This exercise is best done in your hallway. As you walk forward, work to step over the object, continue to walk forward and step over the next object, continuing until you reach the end of the hallway.

ADVANCED WALKING EXERCISES

STEP-UPS AT A FASTER PACE

INTRODUCTION

If you found the step-up exercise in Chapter five a little too easy, this variation is a little more of a challenge. Instead of stepping up with your right leg and then your left slowly, you will step up with your right leg followed by your left leg quickly, and then step down in the same manner. A recommendation is to use a shallow aerobic step on the floor if you have one, as it is about five inches tall, and place it against a wall with a chair beside you for support.

ADVANCED WALKING EXERCISES
AEROBIC CHALLENGE

INTRODUCTION

This aerobic challenge will combine some of the exercises you learned earlier in this chapter. Make sure to have space so you can move!

INSTRUCTIONS

1. Starting in the middle, walk forward for four counts as you did in the heel-to-toe touches. Your left heel will tap first, and then lead you backward. Repeat this pattern four times before returning to the center.
2. Next, move into the lateral step move. Step out with your right leg, then your left.
3. Step in with your right, and then your left. Repeat the pattern four times. Afterwards, do 8-10 high knees on each leg.
4. Lastly, do 10 heel touches on each leg, before switching sides and starting on the left.

Do the challenge twice! You will get a great mental challenge, but also bring in some daily steps! If you get mixed up, don't worry about it, you can try again.

CHAPTER SEVEN

TARGETING SPECIFIC AREAS OF THE BODY

Exercises don't always focus on using one specific muscle, but isolating will target one specific area, which will contribute to strengthening the other muscles in the area.

Focusing on specific areas of the body is especially beneficial if you are looking to rehabilitate an injury or a muscular imbalance.

LEG STRENGTHENING EXERCISES

Our legs have some of the most prominent muscle groups in our entire body. They are the foundation holding us up, much like a foundation holds up a house. When you focus on your legs, you are more likely to improve and support healthier movement in your daily life, such as walking or standing. In addition, a strong lower body helps you avoid injuries, and manage your arthritis, osteoarthritis, heart disease, and diabetes.

In addition, focusing on one leg at a time helps your body's alignment to correct imbalances, and focus on mobility and flexibility, since you are using both sides of your body equally. This will ensure that your dominant leg does not overcompensate your non-dominant side.

EASY LEG STRENGTHENING EXERCISES

HIP EXTENSIONS

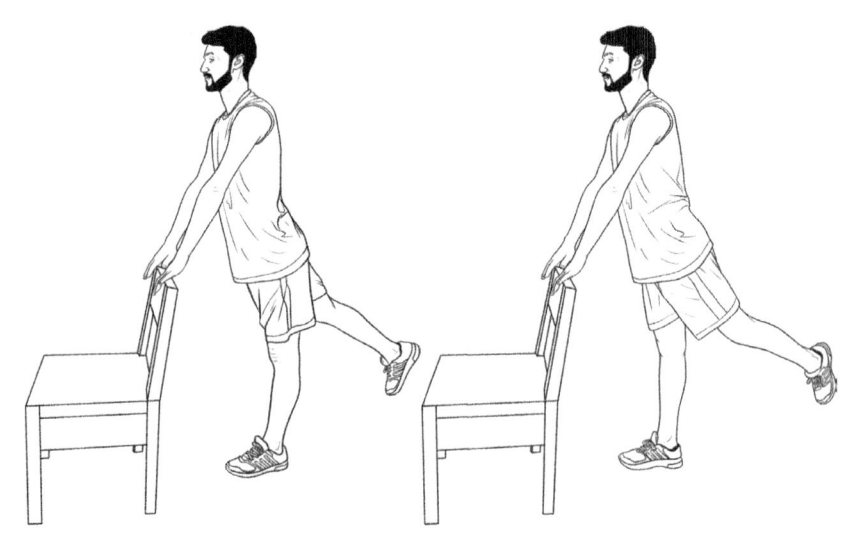

INTRODUCTION

Moving your legs requires the best functionality in your hips. By targeting and strengthening your hip flexors in hip extensions, you will work on stabilizing your pelvis, and feel more vigorous as you walk. In this exercise, you'll target your adductor Magnus which changes its length based on the angle of your hip. You will also work on your gluteal group, which is responsible for moving your hips and thighs. The hip extensions will also focus on your hamstrings, which help support your glutes, particularly when moving from sitting to standing and vice versa.

For this exercise, you will need to use a chair for support.

INSTRUCTIONS

1. Stand behind the chair with your hands placed on the backrest.
2. Keep your legs straight and knees soft.
3. Slowly bring your right leg out behind you with your foot just a few inches above the ground. Your toes should be facing the floor in a relaxed state.
4. Bring your right foot in to repeat on your left side.

Repeat this exercise for 8-12 repetitions in two to three sets. One repetition is counted as both legs moving outwards.

EASY LEG STRENGTHENING EXERCISES
LUNGES

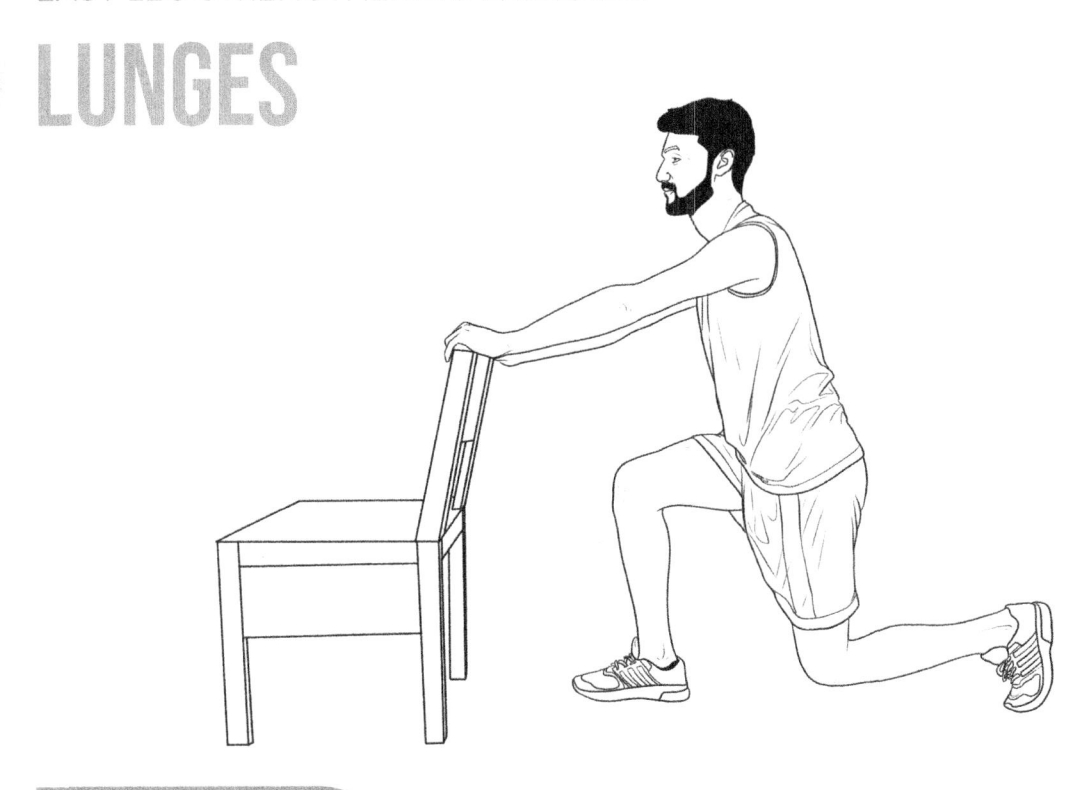

INTRODUCTION

Lunges are one of the best exercises for any age. However, lunges are especially important for seniors, as they will help target various muscles, including the inner thighs, that might have weakened over time. You may use a chair for stability if you like; make sure to have it at the side of your body.

INSTRUCTIONS

1. Begin by standing with your legs hip distance apart.
2. Step forward with your right leg pressing your weight into the heel of your foot.
3. Relax your shoulders, and engage your core.
   Begin lowering your knees until they are at 90 degrees. Remember to listen to your body; if 90 degrees is too far, only lunge as far as is comfortable.
4. Push your weight into your front heel as you straighten upwards. Repeat on the right leg for 8-12 sets before switching sides.

You will repeat this exercise for two to three sets in total.

MEDIUM TO ADVANCED LEG STRENGTHENING EXERCISES

REVERSE LUNGES

INTRODUCTION

Unlike the classic lunge that activates your quads to do most of the work, the reverse lunge will challenge your glutes to take over with the motion as they stretch. What is also excellent about reverse lunges is that you will step backward, which we don't do every single day, thus challenging your brain to focus on where to disperse your weight to keep your balance and body upright. Again, you will need a chair for stability in this exercise.

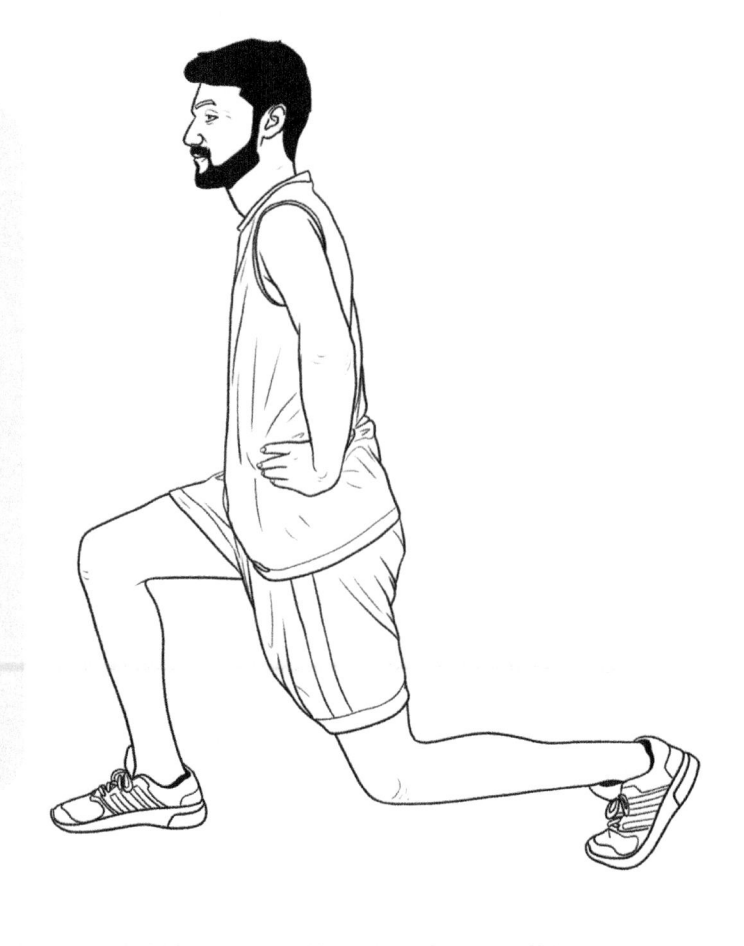

INSTRUCTIONS

1. Facing the back of the chair, take a step back with your right leg while simultaneously bending your knees to the floor. Try to get to 90 degrees if you can.
2. Pressing your weight into your left heel, step forward with your right, and repeat on the other side.

↻ Make sure with each reverse lunge that your body remains upright by engaging your core muscles, and that your knee is not buckling inwards or going over your toes.

Repeat this exercise for two to three sets, 8-12 repetitions. A repetition is each leg going into the reverse lunge.

MEDIUM TO ADVANCED LEG STRENGTHENING EXERCISES
MODIFIED SQUATS

INTRODUCTION

Regardless of age, squats are one of the most beneficial exercises we can add to any workout routine as the multi-movement targets your hips, quads, glutes, hamstrings, and lower back muscles. However, not everyone can perform a squat, and assistance is needed. You will grab a chair and place it against the wall with your hands on the backrest for the modified squats. This is how you perform a modified squat safely.

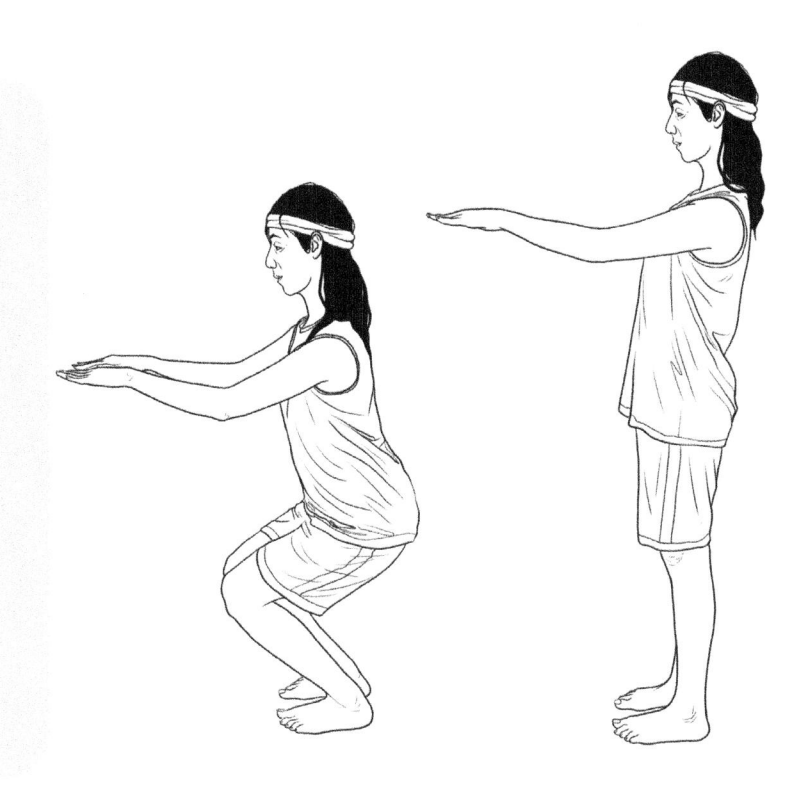

INSTRUCTIONS

1. Standing behind the chair, take a step back so your arms are straight, and your body is centered.
2. Position your legs hip-width apart, with your toes pointed forward.
Press your weight into your heels.
3. As you bend your knees to move toward the floor, envision that you will sit in an invisible chair, stopping at 90 degrees if you can. Ensure that your knees are not going over your toes, and your knees are not collapsing inwards.
Press your weight into your heels as you return to your standing position.

Helpful tip: Make sure not to put all your weight into the chair. Your goal is to challenge your balance as you squat down and up.
Repeat this exercise 8-12 times for two to three sets.

MEDIUM TO ADVANCED LEG STRENGTHENING EXERCISES

SINGLE LEG CROSS-BODY PUNCHES

INTRODUCTION

As we age, our ability to execute tasks efficiently declines, which includes agility and action time. Therefore, by working on this dynamic exercise, not only will it add an aerobic challenge, you will be able to work on improving your hand-eye coordination too.

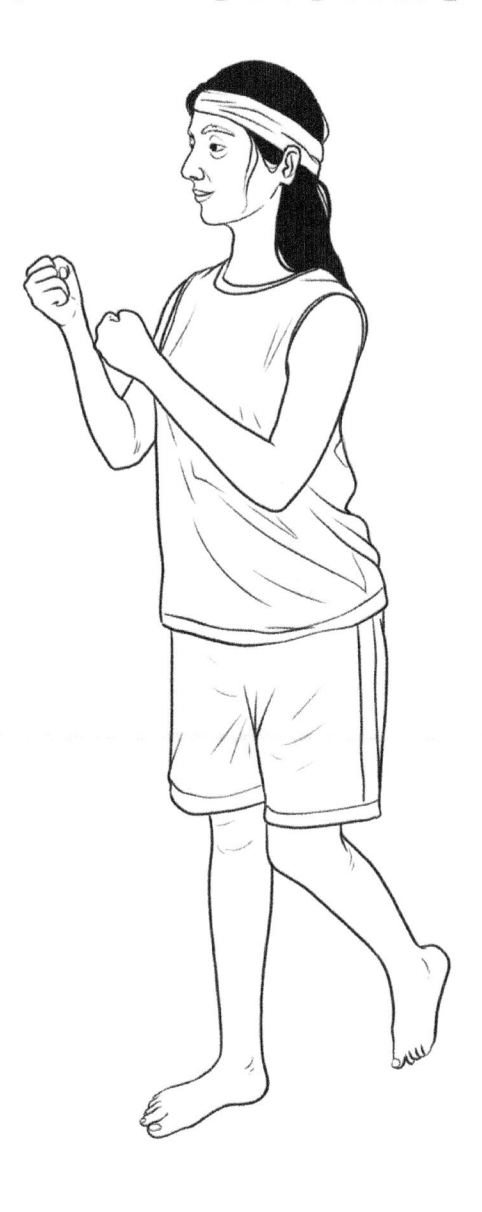

INSTRUCTIONS

1. Start standing on your right leg, and lifting your left a few inches off the ground. Slow punch your left arm to your right by twisting your spine.
2. Repeat the same motion with your left while remaining on your right leg.
3. Lower your left foot down to switch sides.

↻ Repeat each side five times.

CORE STRENGTHENING EXERCISES

For some, when they picture a core, they might vision a fitness model on the front of a fitness magazine. However, this section in our bodies contains all of the muscles to assist with everything else in our body, making it crucial to maintain.

How long it will take to strengthen your core depends on how strong it is to start. To make it stronger and maintain it, you should make core strengthening exercises a part of your weekly routine at least two to three times a week. As you strengthen these groups of muscles, you will improve your coordination, stability, and balance, to help you with everything you enjoy doing daily.

In addition, having a solid core helps to improve your posture and reduce back pain. Our core muscles are responsible for keeping us upright. When they are weaker, we are more likely to slouch, and cause pain in our back, which can set us up for injury.

If you want to continue chasing your grandkids in a game of tag, or maybe enjoy playing badminton, keeping your body in working shape is essential, and a strong core can help you in that direction.

EASY CORE STRENGTHENING EXERCISES

SEATED HALF ROLL-BACKS

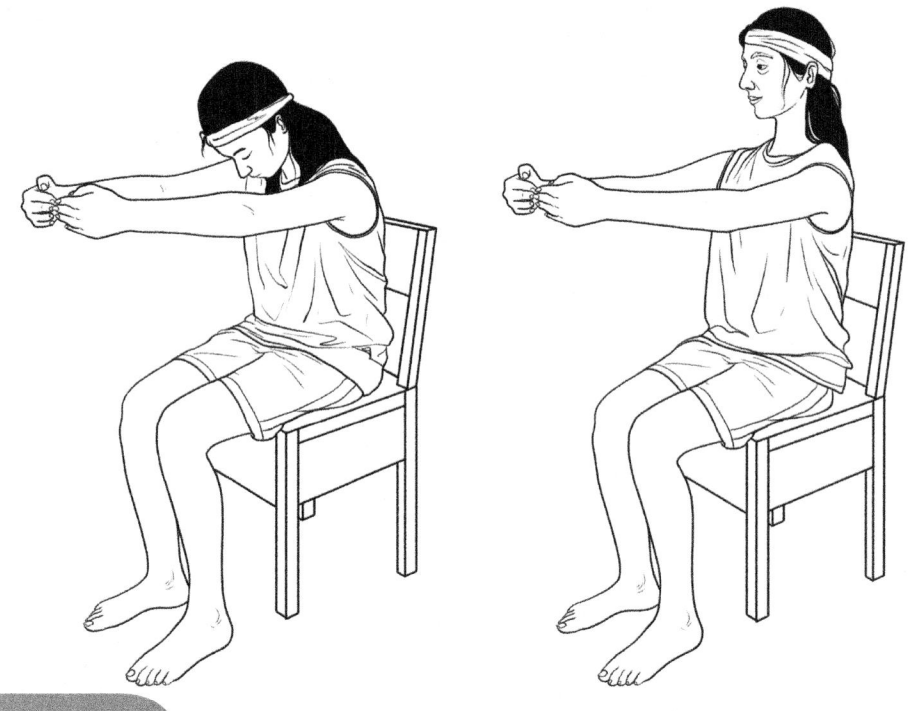

INTRODUCTION

The seated half roll-back is a pilates move that helps to strengthen your core, and make your spine a little more flexible. As you roll your spine, you will activate your lower abs to keep the movement slow. You might even feel a little tension release as it stretches a little bit of your upper back. So grab your chair, and let's get started!

INSTRUCTIONS

1. For this exercise, you will need to sit in your chair. Your feet need to be flat on the floor.
2. Bring your arms up in front of you, with your fingers interlocked to form a circle. Begin to round your back by scooping in your abs as far as is comfortable.
3. Think of it as ife you are hollowing out your stomach and creating a 'C' shape. Hold for 30 seconds, then slowly roll back to your starting position.

↻ Repeat this exercise eight times.

EASY CORE STRENGTHENING EXERCISES

SEATED FORWARD ROLL-UPS

INTRODUCTION

The seated forward roll-ups are a full variation of the half roll-ups. This exercise will further help your spine's flexibility for better functionality throughout your daily tasks.

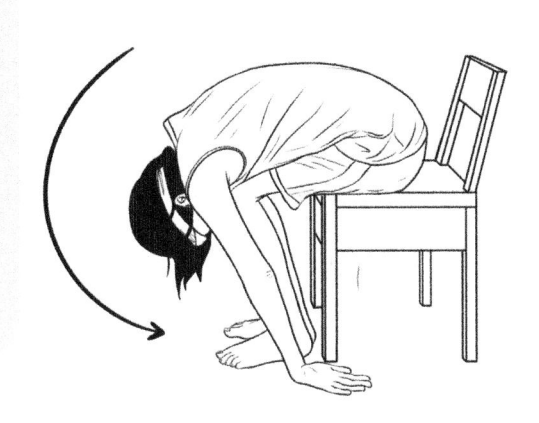

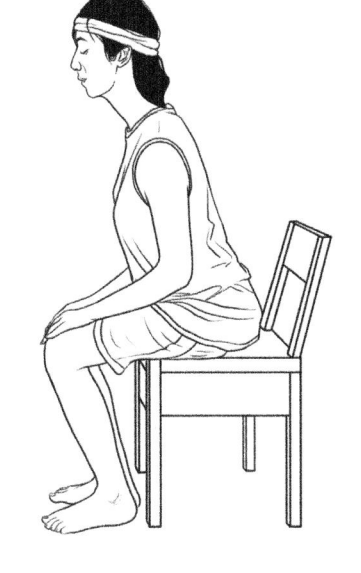

INSTRUCTIONS

1. Sitting in your chair, extend your legs in front of you. Your legs should be in a diagonal from your hip, with your ankle flexed, and your toes facing the ceiling.
2. Inhale as you bring your arms out in front of you. Engage your core to maintain an upright position.
3. As you exhale, bring your chin to your chest.
4. Hollow your stomach as you roll your torso up and over, as if you are bending over a beam. Make sure your legs remain straight, and your core is engaged as you reach down towards your toes as far as you can go.
   When you have reached as far as possible, inhale and begin to roll back up bone by bone to the starting position.

↻ Repeat the movement slowly five more times.

EASY CORE STRENGTHENING EXERCISES

SEATED SIDE BENDS

INTRODUCTION

Doing a side bend challenges your imbalances to correct themselves by lengthening your abs and hips, while improving your spine's flexibility. This fun move also helps stretch your muscles between your ribs, since they can get tight and short due to poor posture and hours of sitting.

Side bends are also great for helping the flexibility in your ribs, making the movement awesome if you have breathing issues since it can open your lungs. You might even find some relief from respiratory conditions such as allergies.

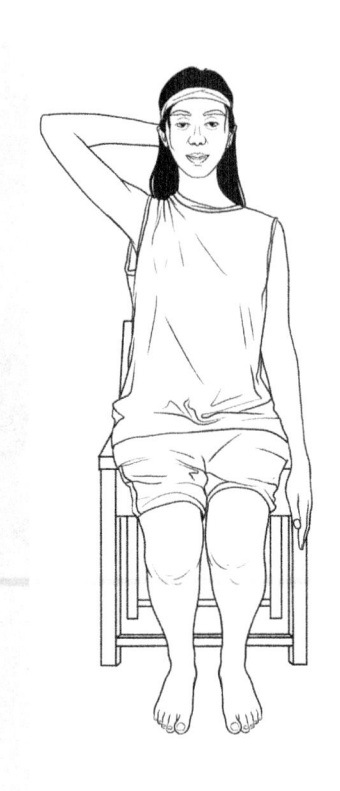

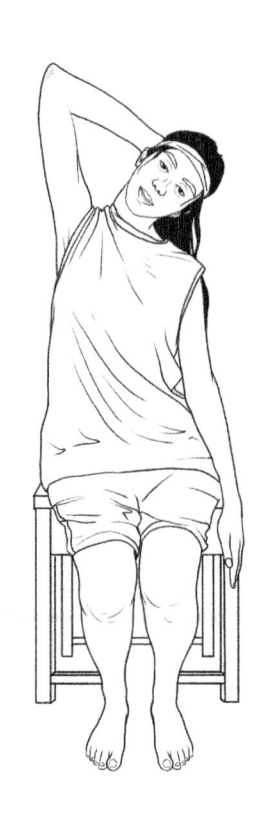

INSTRUCTIONS

1. Sit in your chair with your feet flat on the ground. Ensure to maintain a lengthened spine.
2. Put your right hand on the right side of your head, while allowing your left arm to hang at the side, and inhale.
3. As you exhale, bend sideways at your waist to lower your left arm to the floor. Make sure to keep your chest open by pulling your elbow back.
Inhale to uncurl the bend and repeat.

For this exercise, do two to three sets with 8-12 repetitions. One set includes both sides.

MEDIUM TO ADVANCED CORE STRENGTHENING EXERCISES

SUPERMAN

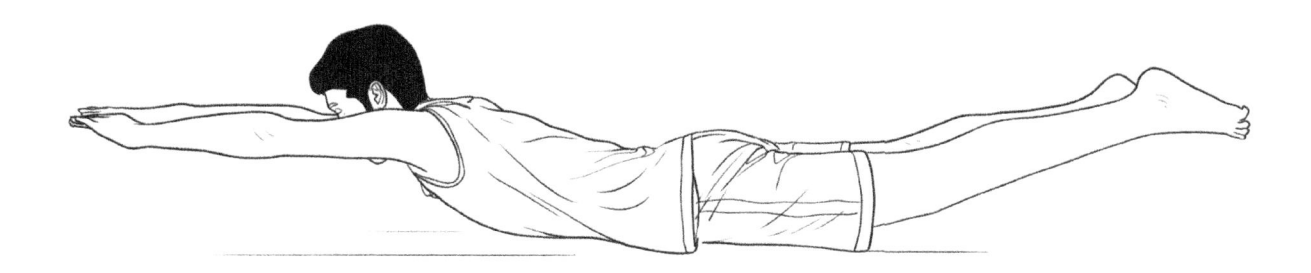

INTRODUCTION

For this exercise, let's be a superhero, as Superman will help improve your lumbar and hip extensions for better stability. This is one of the core exercises you can perform daily, as it can also help strengthen your lower back, and prevent back pain. For this exercise, you'll be lying on the floor. If getting up and down from the floor is difficult for you, skipping this exercise is recommended.

INSTRUCTIONS

1. On the floor, lie down on your stomach with your legs extended out behind you, and your arms extended over your head. Keep your knees soft. Your shoulders should be down as well.
2. Inhale to draw your abs toward your spine, creating a gap between your stomach and the floor.
3. As you exhale, activate your abs and glutes to bring your arms and legs off the floor together, with your gaze on the floor.
Inhale to return to the starting position.

Repeat this exercise 8-10 times.

MEDIUM TO ADVANCED CORE STRENGTHENING EXERCISES

MODIFIED PLANKS

INTRODUCTION

Planks are one of the best exercises you can do in a workout because they can help improve your posture and stability. Your core is essential to keeping your spine in alignment, and with good posture, you are less likely to develop injuries when your weight is improperly distributed.

If you have an issue with your back, planks can also help reduce back pain as you build up the muscles in your abs. You will also improve your coordination.

For the modified planks, you will do the exercise using the wall for support.

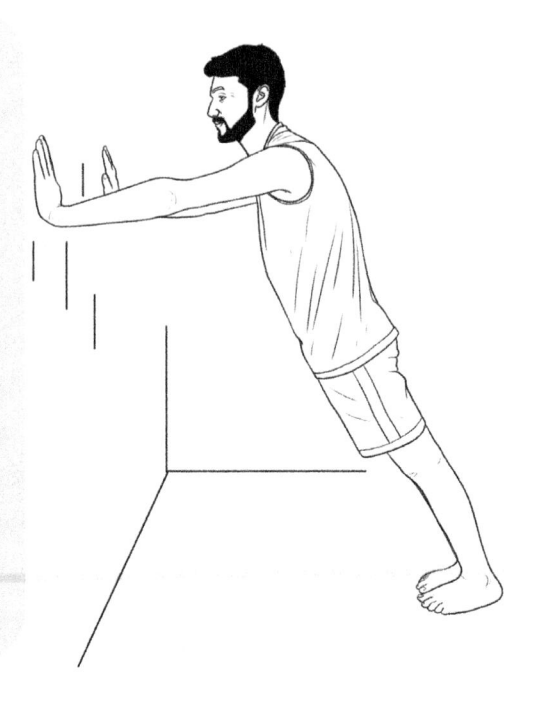

INSTRUCTIONS

1. To set up, place both hands shoulder-width apart at chest height. Make sure your arms are soft at the elbows.
2. Shift your feet back so that you are in a diagonal position. Your body should replicate a straight line from your head to heel. It is essential to ensure your buttocks are not too high in the air, and your back is not arched.
3. Stay in the position for 30 seconds, or whatever is most comfortable for you. Bring your feet forward to reset, before moving back into a plank.

Repeat the exercise two to three times.

If you want a challenge, try using a chair or an aerobic step, following the same steps above. For safety measures, make sure to put your chair or aerobic step against the wall for stability.

UPPER BODY STRENGTHENING EXERCISES

Upper body exercises have a lasting effect on your independence. Next to walking, using our upper body to reach is one of the other everyday movements we do daily. Therefore, building strength in our shoulders, arms, and upper back allows us to easily reach for items on that high shelf, or lift our grandchildren, while maintaining our balance in the movements.

Easy Upper Body Strengthening Exercises

For these exercises, a couple of cans of soup will do for light weights. Each activity will be repeated in two to three sets 8-12 times. Each set counts when both sides have been completed.

EASY UPPER BODY STRENGTHENING EXERCISES

BICEP CURLS

INTRODUCTION

The bicep curl is one of the most known weight-training exercises to work your upper arm muscles. They are a set of muscles you use daily without even thinking about when you go to pick something up, like your groceries or your laundry.

This exercise is an elbow exercise as the repetitive bending will help strengthen your upper arm and make lifting objects much more effortless. You can do this exercise either standing up or seated.

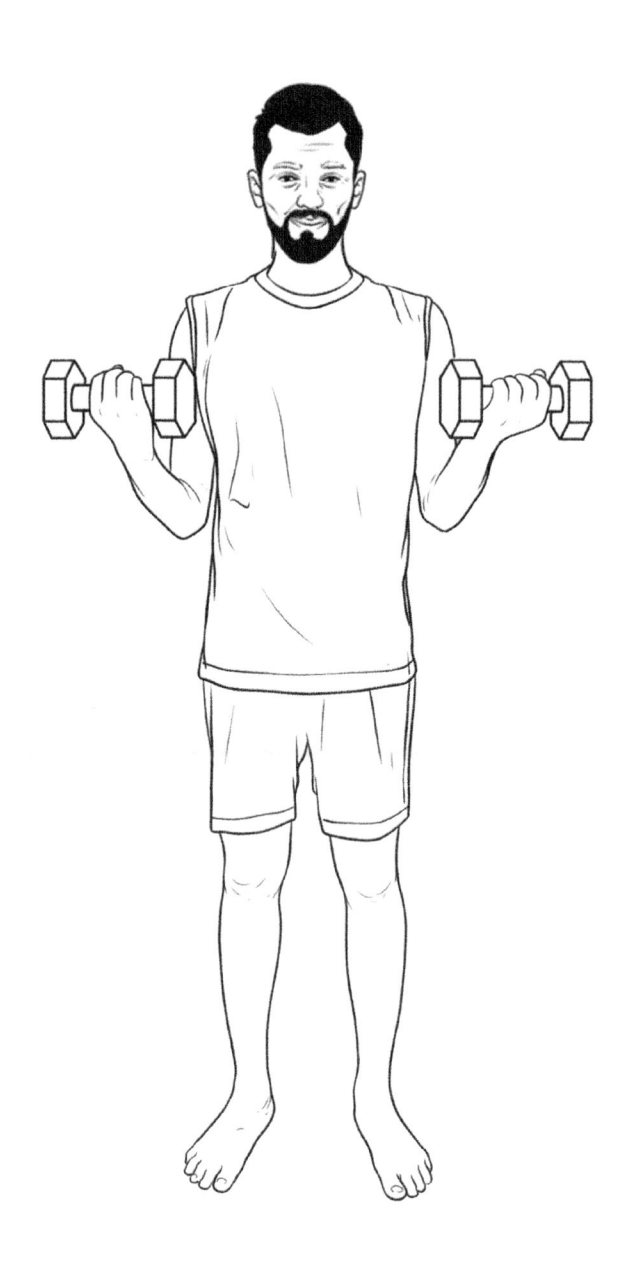

INSTRUCTIONS

1. Hold the weights in your hands with your arms by your side. Your palms need to be facing outwards.
2. Inhale and bend your elbows to bring your weight up to your shoulder. Exhale as you lower the weight.

↻ Try alternating sides with each lift if you want to challenge your stability and balancing technique.

EASY UPPER BODY STRENGTHENING EXERCISES

TRICEPS KICKBACKS

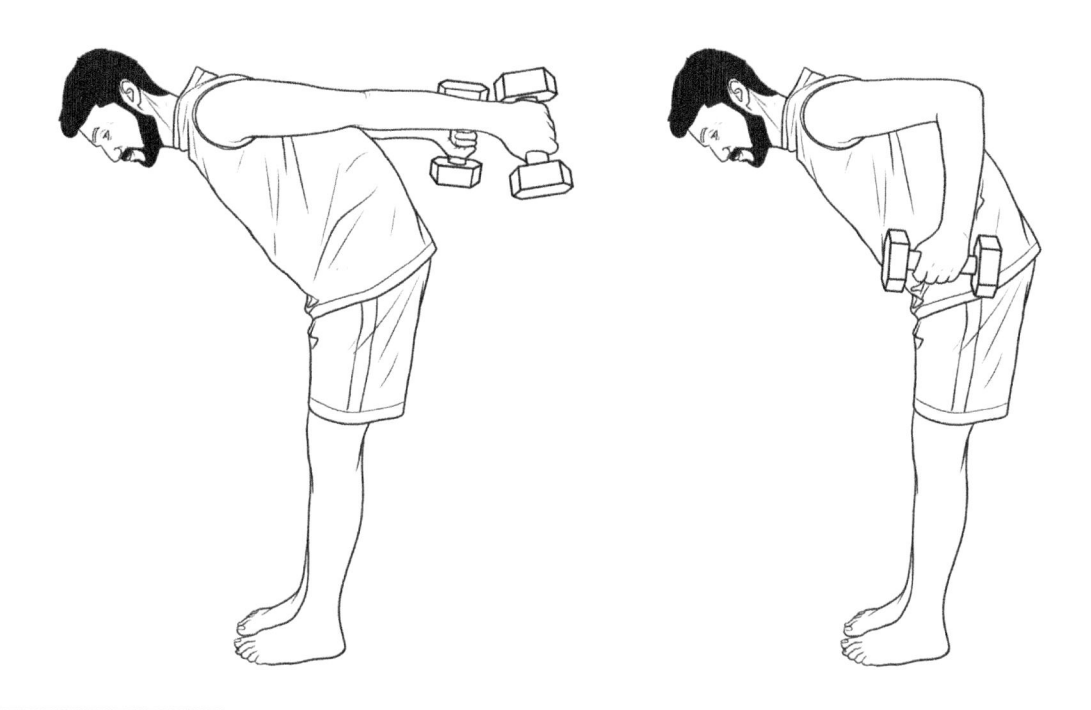

INTRODUCTION

Triceps kickbacks give you better power and strength to lift yourself from a chair with armrests or from your bed. Our triceps also help extend our arm when you reach your hand above your head to get something from high up.

When doing this exercise, keep your elbows high for the backwards motion. You might want to use the back of a chair for support, as you will be bent over slightly.

INSTRUCTIONS

1. Hold your weight in your right hand when leaning over your chair, or place your left hand on your left thigh for support.
2. Extend your arm back behind you as far as it is comfortable.
3. Bring your arm back in.

MEDIUM TO ADVANCED UPPER BODY STRENGTHENING EXERCISES

DIAGONAL INWARD SHOULDER RAISE

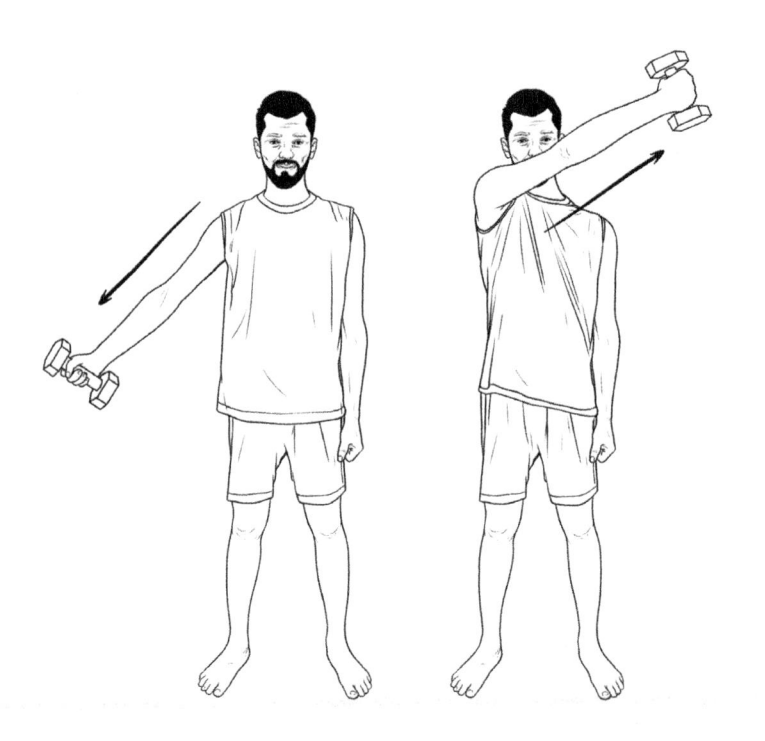

INTRODUCTION

The diagonal inward shoulder raise will help maintain a strong upper body, so you can easily lift your groceries, do laundry, open doors and windows, and put the dishes away. In addition, in a diagonal position, the muscles in your shoulder and upper arm will strengthen better to improve overall functionality, while performing those daily tasks. You'll also be able to increase your mobility for a better arm swing when you walk, or when you are marching on the spot for some quick cardio. This movement can be done either seated or standing.

INSTRUCTIONS

1. Sitting or standing, have the weight in your right hand, and your arm placed by your side. Turn your walk outwards.
2. Inhale as you lift your arm across your body to your left shoulder. Your palm will turn inward as you pull the weight up and across you. Move slowly and controlled as you lift the weight.
3. Exhale as you return to the starting position.

MEDIUM TO ADVANCED UPPER BODY STRENGTHENING EXERCISES

DIAGONAL OUTWARD SHOULDER RAISE

INTRODUCTION

Like the diagonal inward shoulder raise, the outwards motion in this exercise will help you with reaching overhead into those high shelves. However, the outwards motion also helps you reach into low pantries, or open stubborn cupboard doors. You should also be able to sweep or mop your house quickly. Again, you can sit or stand for this exercise.

INSTRUCTIONS

1. Sitting or standing, place the weight in your right hand, and have it crossed over to your left side. Your palm needs to be facing inward this time.
2. Inhale and lift your arm across your body, ending just past shoulder height, or whichever is most comfortable for you.
3. Exhale to bring your weight back down to the starting position.

MEDIUM TO ADVANCED UPPER BODY STRENGTHENING EXERCISES

OVERHEAD PRESS

INTRODUCTION

This is one of the more demanding exercises you can do to strengthen your shoulders. However, your stability will improve with this exercise as you learn to reach overhead safely. In addition, your shoulder joints' mobility will be strengthened too.

As this exercise is a little more advanced than the others, take this exercise slow, and don't use any weight. Also, only do eight repetitions per set until you are more comfortable doing up to 12.

INSTRUCTIONS

1. Stand with your feet shoulder distance apart, your hands at chest level, and your palms facing forward.
2. Inhale and raise your arms together straight up. Your upper arms should frame your head.
3. Exhale and lower your arms to the starting position.

STRETCHING EXERCISES

Stretching allows us to move more freely, as tension releases from our joints, while also helping improve our posture. You should be stretching every time you work out, but you also have great benefits when you get up in the morning, or are getting ready, because it will help with circulation, control your muscles and how they move, and improve your balance and coordination. Stretching for 10 minutes twice a day is recommended.

STRETCHING EXERCISES
NECK STRETCH

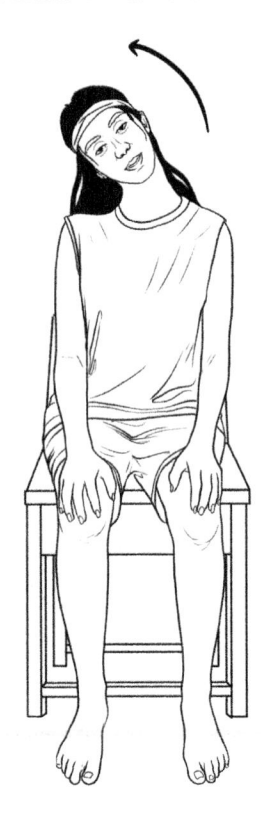

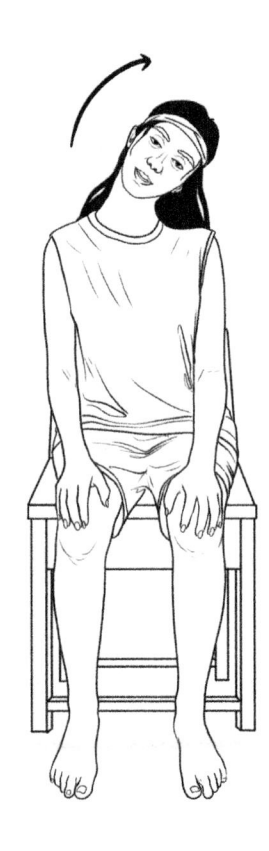

INTRODUCTION

Doing a neck stretch allows you to maintain mobility in your neck for posture, and turning your head while driving or walking. This can be done either sitting or standing.

INSTRUCTIONS

1. Start by tilting your chin to your chest to stretch the back of your neck. Hold for 15 to 20 seconds.
2. Slowly bring your head back up.
   To stretch your right side, tilt your head to the left, and hold for 15 to 20 seconds.
3. Slowly bring your head back to the center, and repeat on the other side.

↻ Repeat the exercise three to five times.

STRETCHING EXERCISES

SHOULDER AND UPPER ARM STRETCH

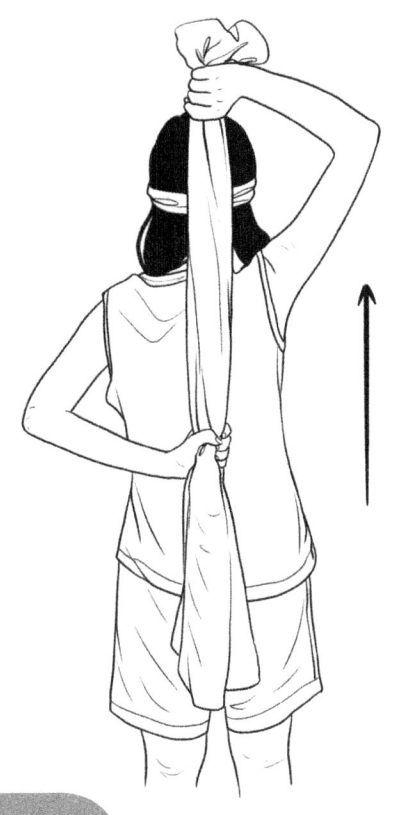

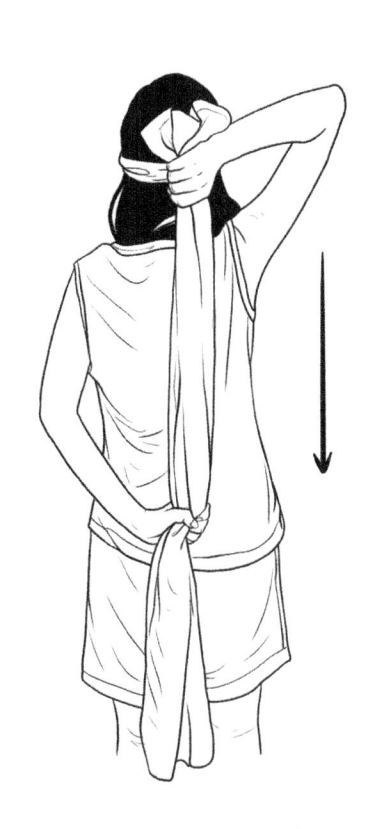

INTRODUCTION

Although working out your arms is important so you can easily lift things, making sure they are mobile with stretching is equally important. For this stretch, grab a kitchen towel.

INSTRUCTIONS

1. Stand with your legs shoulder-width apart. Hold your towel in your right hand, draping it on your right shoulder, so it goes down your back.
2. Grab the other end of your towel with your left hand, and pull down until you feel a comfortable stretch.
3. Hold for 15 to 20 seconds, and then switch sides.

STRETCHING EXERCISES

QUADRICEPS STRETCH

INTRODUCTION

Our quadriceps are located in the front of our upper leg. They are our biggest muscles, and are responsible for walking and standing. Remember the foundation of a house? Your quadriceps can be compared to that. You can do this lying down. However, standing challenges your balancing capabilities. Use a chair, wall, table, or countertop for stability.

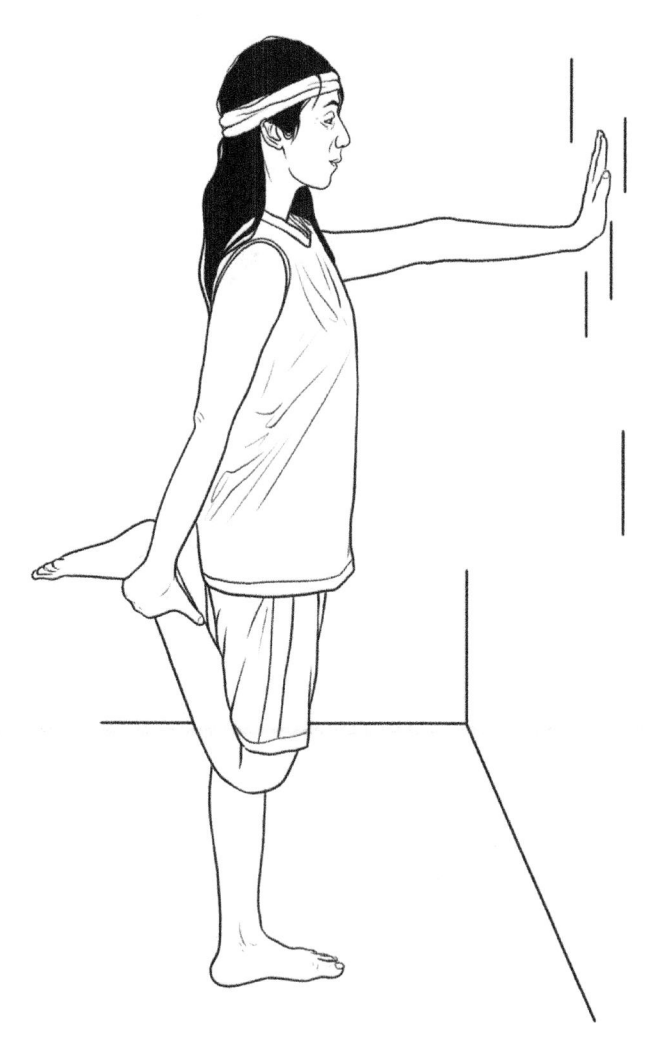

INSTRUCTIONS

1. Begin with having your supporting chair on your left side. Bend your right knee to bring your foot to your buttocks, catching your ankle with your right hand.
2. Pull your ankle closer to feel the stretch in your quad, only going as far as your body tells you.
3. Hold for 15 to 20 seconds before releasing.
4. Turn to repeat on your left leg.

STRETCHING EXERCISES
HIP STRETCH

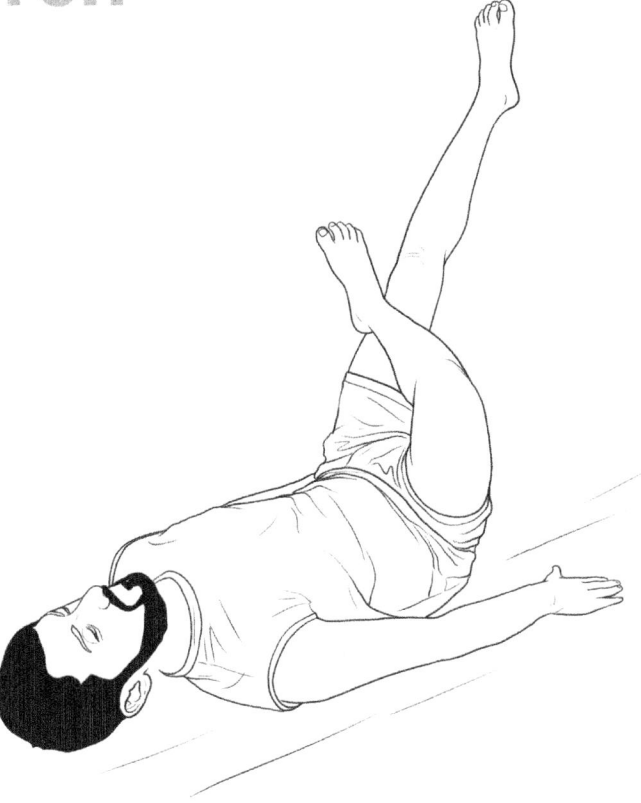

INTRODUCTION

Older adults, particularly women, are known to carry a fair amount of tension in their hips. The tighter your hips are, the less mobility you have, which can result in pain as you walk or use the stairs. Having tight hips can also cause a forward tilt in the pelvis, and cause poor posture or misaligning your head and neck. For this stretch, you are going to lie down on your back. After that, you can lie on your floor or bed.

INSTRUCTIONS

1. Bring your right knee to the side of your body, and rest your foot on top of your opposite leg. Picture the tree pose in yoga.
2. Gently push your right knee down, until you feel a stretch that is comfortable for you.
3. Hold for 15 to 20 seconds before switching sides.

STRETCHING EXERCISES
LOWER BACK STRETCH

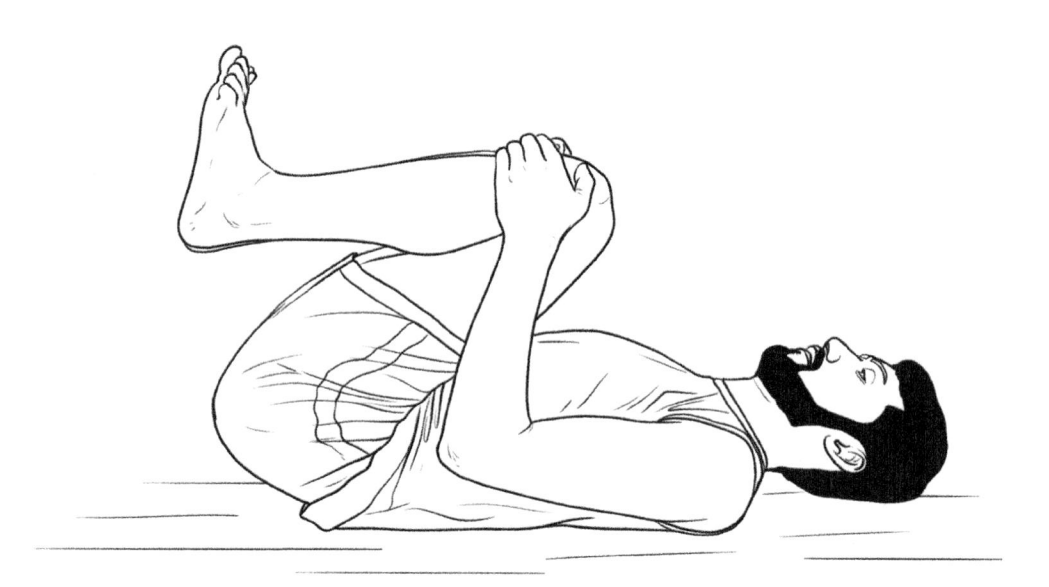

INTRODUCTION

Lower back pain is a common complaint most people have. However, seniors are more prone to lower back pain due to wear and tear in the spinal discs and joints. This is why it is essential to stretch out your back to relieve the tension, and maintain an upright position. You can stretch your lower back by lying on the floor or in bed.

INSTRUCTIONS

1. Lie down with your knees and feet flat on the floor.
   Bring your knees up, and gently hug them to your chest.
2. Twist your torso to the right until you feel a stretch that is comfortable for you.

↻ Hold for 15 to 20 seconds, and then repeat on the other side.

CHAPTER EIGHT
VESTIBULAR EXERCISES

Our vestibular system is one of the oldest sensory systems in our bodies. As the system is responsible for how the central nervous system functions, the vestibular organ helps us detect and control the movement in our environments.

Fay et al. (2004) say that the vestibular system includes brain functions such as "sleep, vision, audition, somatosensation movement, digestion, cognition, learning, and memory."

So what is the vestibular system exactly? Simply put, it is a complex sensory system that helps maintain our balance and spatial orientation. If you have seen a gymnast compete on an impressive horizontal bar or balance beam routine, their ability to stay balanced and be aware of their surroundings is all thanks to the vestibular system.

The vestibular system is found in our inner ear. When something goes wrong, such as a severe ear infection, it can cause you to feel dizzy, experience vertigo, or induce an imbalance. You might even experience blurred vision. There are two types of vestibular balance disorders:

Benign Paroxysmal Positional Vertigo, which is one of the most common causes. This vestibular disorder usually happens when someone makes a quick motion, such as standing too quickly from sitting, or turning over in bed.

A build-up of fluid in the vestibular's labyrinth causes Meniere's Disease. You might feel severely nauseated or dizzy if you have Meniere's Disease.

If you experience problems with your balance, the best advice that I can offer is not to panic. There are ways to overcome dizziness by building up tolerance in your brain, like building muscle strength.

You will know if you need vestibular training if you experience persistent systems, such as those listed, or the following:

- Feeling unsteady
- Woozy
- Lightheaded
- Feeling faint or that you might faint
- Moving sensations

- Spinning
- Swaying

It is important to note that feeling dizzy is not necessarily profound; it can happen to anyone. Have you ever rolled down a hill as a child and felt dizzy? It usually passes quickly. However, if you are experiencing persistent symptoms, it's probably your body telling you something is off. It could be something as simple as a medication's side effects, but it could also be more serious, such as a heart or brain problem. If you are concerned, please reach out to your physician before trying out any of these exercises.

As for the exercises in this chapter, the goal is repetition, so that your brain can learn to handle and directly interpret the stimulation. In addition, it will learn how to adapt to abnormal activity; it's not like you shake your head for several hours a day, but specific movements, especially if you have vestibular issues, can make you feel off.

These exercises listed below are similar to how figure skaters train to avoid becoming dizzy when they spin rapidly. As you work through the exercises, your other goal is to prepare the movement of your eyes to be independent from your head.

EXERCISES TO IMPROVE YOUR VESTIBULAR ORGAN

This might sound crazy, but in this part, you want to spark a dizzy sensation a few times a day to find control in each episode. When you have mastered control over your dizzy spells, try movements that have previously made you feel dizzy, and spend more time on them until your symptoms subside.

How are vestibular exercises meant to work? The purpose is to improve the central nervous system or the brain's compensation for abnormalities or injuries in the vestibular organ. When abnormalities or injuries occur in any section of the system, the brain needs to relearn how to understand the messages it receives from the rest of the body. Doing exercises stimulates the vestibular apparatus to produce information the brain can process more efficiently. Doing these exercises twice per day is recommended, so you can build up vestibular strength.

HEAD EXERCISES
TURNING SIDE TO SIDE

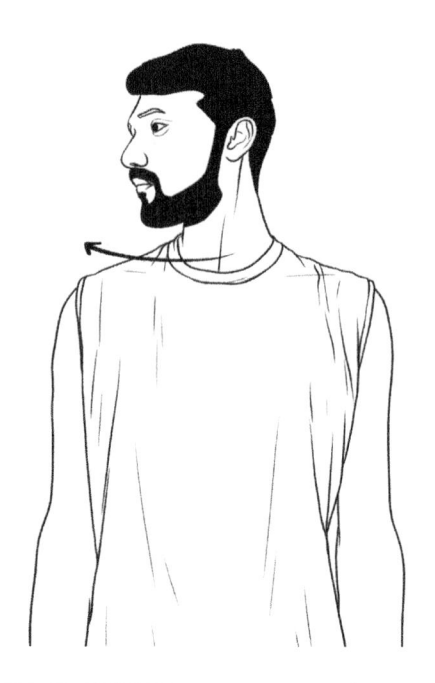

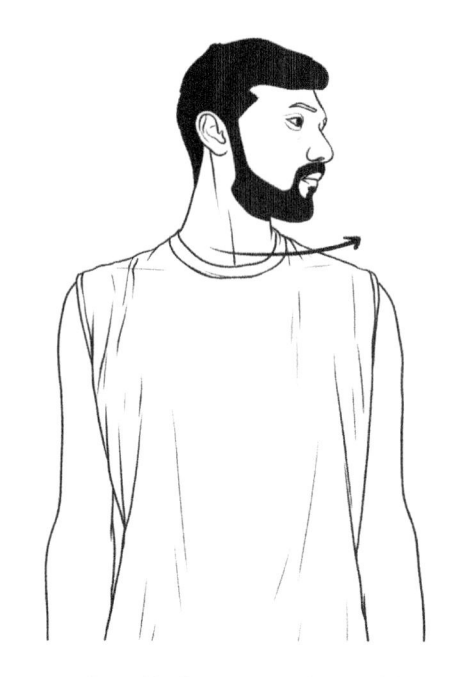

INTRODUCTION

You are going to sit for this exercise. Sitting up, rotate your head to the right and then to the left. You will want to use your eyes to lead your head. Imagine you are watching a tennis or badminton match. The movement of your head should be fast, so that it generates dizzy symptoms, but not so fast that you hurt your neck. So, start slowly and then increase the speed.

INSTRUCTIONS

1. You will want to go back and forth 10 times, and then wait 30 seconds. If your symptoms have not resolved, wait a little longer until they stop. Then, repeat the exercise two more times.
2. When your dizziness begins to improve, try closing your eyes and performing the exercise again. Then, try performing it while standing with your eyes open, and then shut when you have mastered that.

HEAD EXERCISES

STANDING AND THROWING A BALL

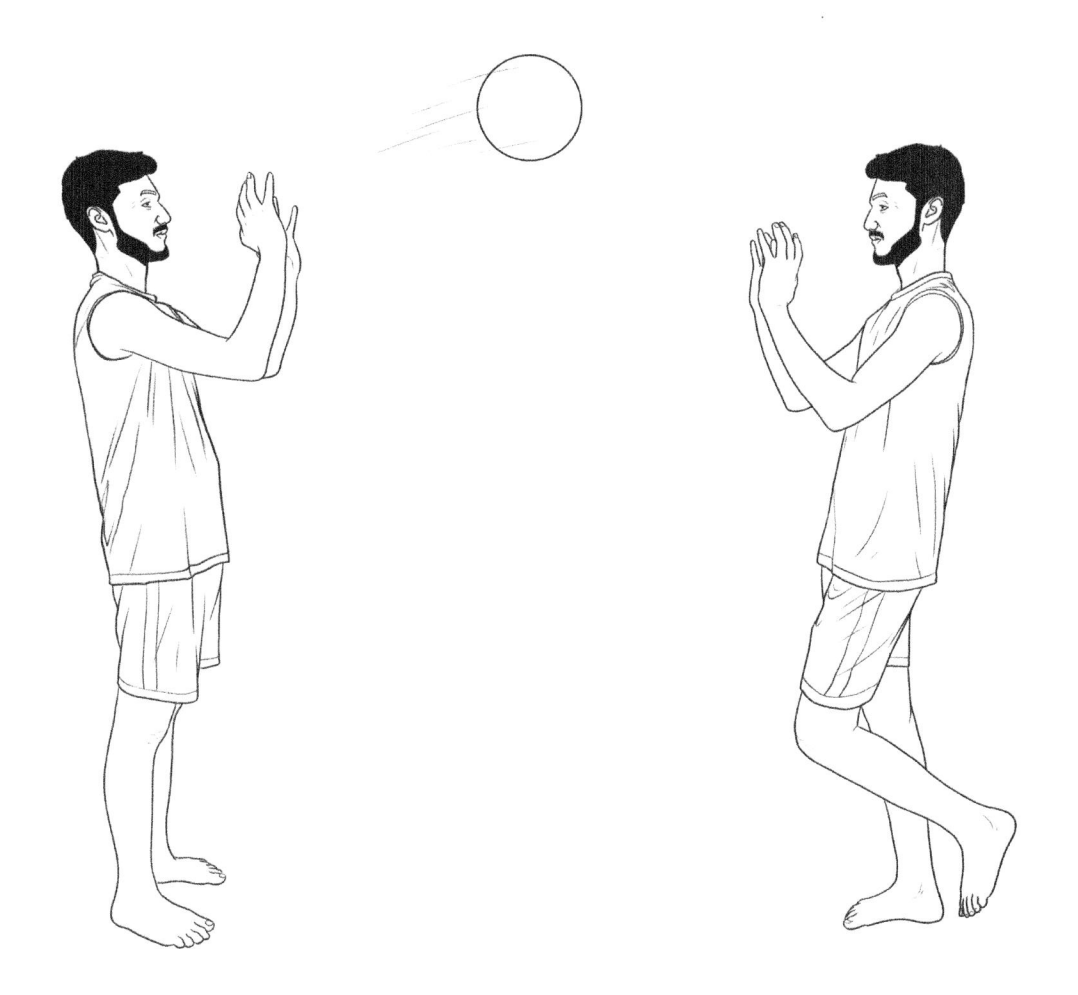

INSTRUCTIONS

1. For this one, you will want a small ball to toss, such as a tennis ball. First, throw the ball from your dominant hand to your non-dominant hand above eye level.

2. Next, throw the ball from hand to hand under one of your knees. For an added challenge, try changing the leg you are tossing under, as if you are creating an infinite symbol.

HEAD EXERCISES

WALKING WHILE TURNING YOUR HEAD

INSTRUCTIONS

1. Using a hallway or an open space, practice walking straight while turning your head right to left with every step. So if you step to your right, you will also look right simultaneously.

2. Continue until you reach the end of your hallway, and then turn around to repeat the process. Walk down your hallway three times in total, back and forth.

3. Let your symptoms resolve before going on to the next part.
   Begin walking in your hallway again, except looking at the ceiling and then the floor.

↻ Repeat three times back and forth in the hallway.

HEAD EXERCISES
LYING DOWN

INSTRUCTIONS

1 Sitting on your bed, quickly lie down on your right side by swinging your feet onto the bed. Lie on the bed for 30 seconds, or until your symptoms stop. Repeat this movement three times before changing to your left side.

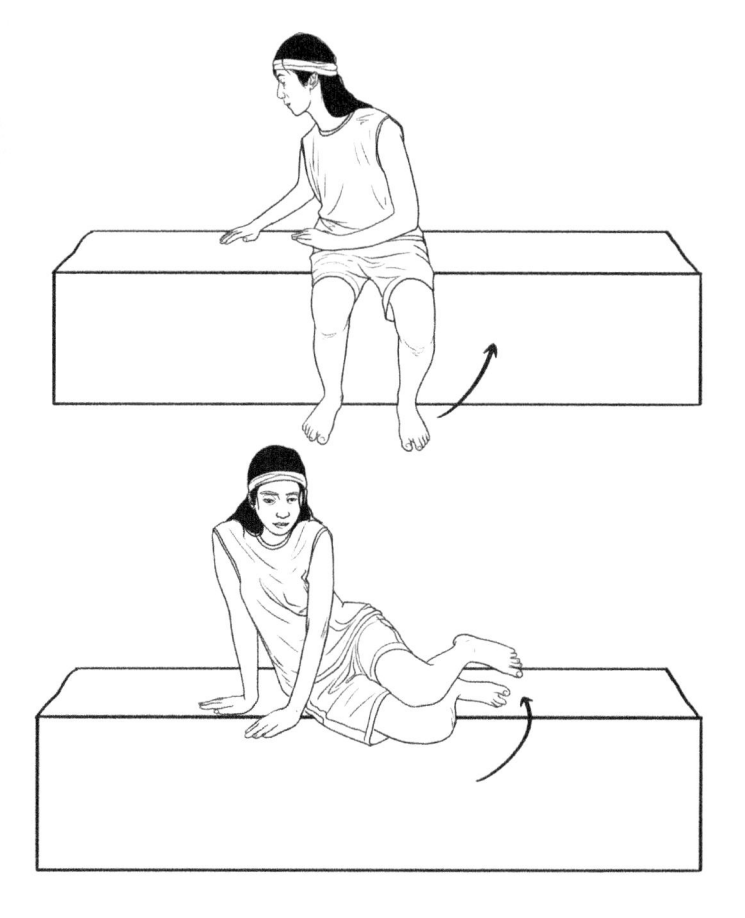

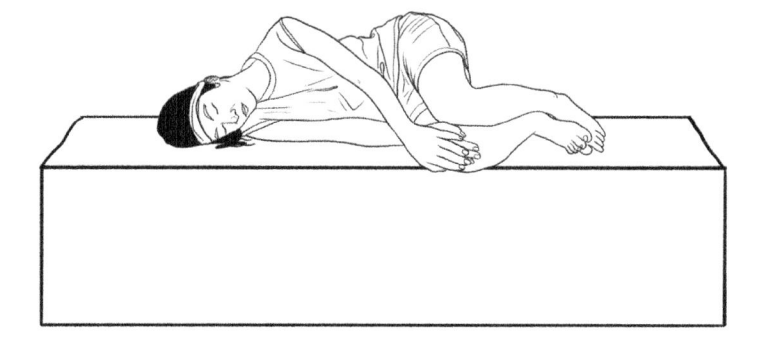

HEAD EXERCISES
GAZE STABILIZATION

INTRODUCTION

Before you begin this exercise, here are some pointers to help you get the most out of gaze stabilization:

Choose a target that is in focus

Perform the activity with a little head movement

You can increase the speed of your head's motion so long as your target is focused

If you wear glasses or contact lenses, be sure you are wearing them while performing this exercise

INSTRUCTIONS

1. For this exercise, keep your eyes fixed on a non-moving object in your hand, or on a wall about three to ten feet away. Move your head from side to side for 30 seconds as if you are shaking your head. Stop and wait for your symptoms to resolve, and then repeat three more times from side to side.
2. Next, you will move your head up and down, as if you are nodding for 30 seconds. Stop to let your symptoms resolve before continuing.
3. It is recommended to do this exercise three times a day. You may not notice it, but this head movement is something we tend to do frequently throughout our day when answering questions.

You might want to progress to standing and working on gaze stabilization as you improve the exercise. The closer your feet are, the harder it will be.

CHAPTER NINE

EXERCISING WITH A PARTNER

There are many benefits to exercising with a partner. You are likely to feel more motivated to work out with someone else, and it is a fun opportunity to engage in some healthy competition too.

Also, as we get older, sometimes it feels easier to stay home, and skip workout days, when you typically exercise by yourself. At least with a partner, you are likely to have more accountability if you plan to go on a walk, or attend an exercise class, because you know your workout friend is counting on you to be there.

You're likely to challenge yourself more when you work with someone instead of alone. A psychological phenomenon called the Kohler Effect somewhat captures how someone's influence can motivate others to push themselves harder. Some research has found that this exciting phenomenon has at least two causes: the "process of social comparison," and "the effects of individual members being indispensable to the group" (Kerr, 2016). For example, when someone is exercising with a partner or within a group, and can see others performing better than they are, it can be "enough to boost an individual's efforts" (Kerr, 2016), and thus, challenge the person to increase their performance goal. Those members challenging the individual would be the indispensable factor in this scenario.

Doing the same activities can feel redundant and probably a little boring, leading to a decrease in motivation. With an exercise partner, however, you can get a little inspiration, and try something new such as outdoor yoga, hiking on a new trail, kayaking, or canoeing… The list is endless on what you can do! Also, if the activity is new to you or both of you, you will likely feel more confident and comfortable trying it when you can face the challenge together.

Lastly, as a senior, having a workout buddy or group is also a great way to gain social interactions!

SAFETY NOTES WHEN EXERCISING WITH A PARTNER

When working out with your friend, always communicate with them about any aches or pains you might be experiencing. In addition, be sure to slow down or stop if you need to. The goal is to have fun, and not injure or further injure yourself or your partner.

Exercises You Can Do With a Partner

There are a lot of activities you can do with a friend or within a group! This section will list some ideas for what you can do with a partner.

EXERCISES YOU CAN DO WITH A PARTNER

BACK ROWS WITH A RESISTANCE BAND

INTRODUCTION

Back rows help strengthen your upper back, while working various muscles in your arms. For this exercise, you'll need an open-ended resistance band which you can find on Amazon, or your local fitness store.

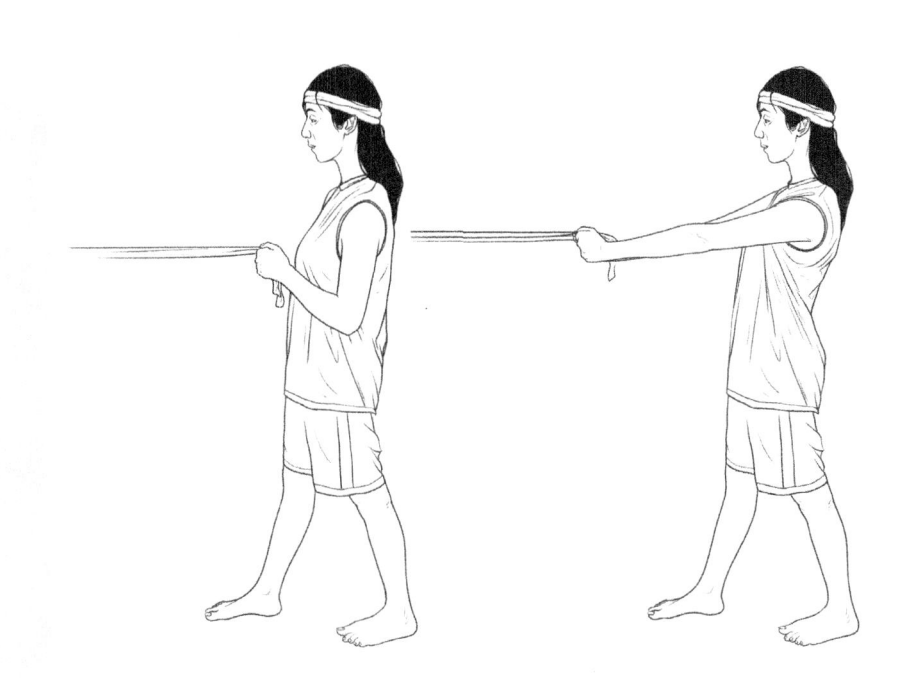

INSTRUCTIONS

1. Holding the ends of your resistance band, stand and face your partner about a foot apart. Your stance needs to be just a little wider than your hips.
2. Next, you and your partner need to step back with one of your legs, to have a staggered stance.
3. Both need to lengthen your spine and tilt your hips forward to avoid hollowing out your back while engaging your core.
4. The supporting partner will then grab the folded end of the resistance band.
5. The partner doing the exercise will then take the ends in each hand.
Inhale as you pull back on the resistance band, pulling your shoulder blades together.
6. Exhale as you release.
7. Repeat 8-12 times and then switch.

↻ You and your partner should do at least two to three sets each.

EXERCISES YOU CAN DO WITH A PARTNER

NECK EXERCISE

INTRODUCTION

The neck exercise helps strengthen your neck muscles to prevent any strains. For this exercise, you will need a chair.

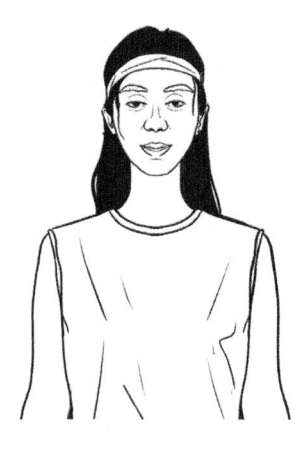

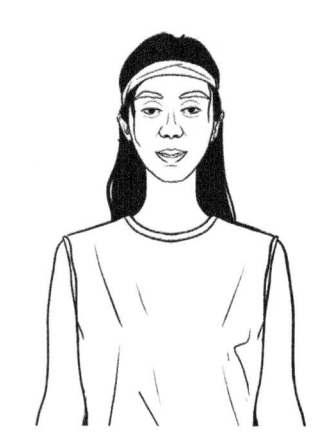

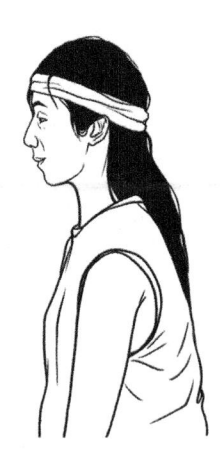

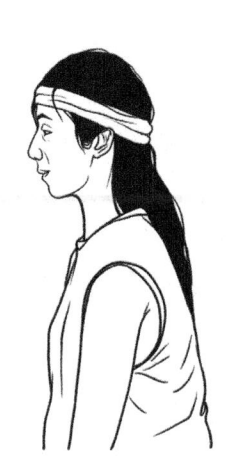

INSTRUCTIONS

1. Sit up straight in your chair with your chin slightly tucked.
   With your partner standing behind you, have them place their hands on either side of your head.
2. Keeping your head straight, gently shift your head to the right to press against your partner's hand, and hold for 10 seconds before returning to the starting position.
3. Repeat the movement on the left.

For this exercise, do five repetitions on each side before switching with your partner.

EXERCISES YOU CAN DO WITH A PARTNER
PARTNER PUSHES

INTRODUCTION

If you and your workout friend want to work on your core strength while maintaining balance, partner pushes are a great unilateral exercise to challenge these areas. In addition, it will improve your chest, tricep, and shoulder strength.

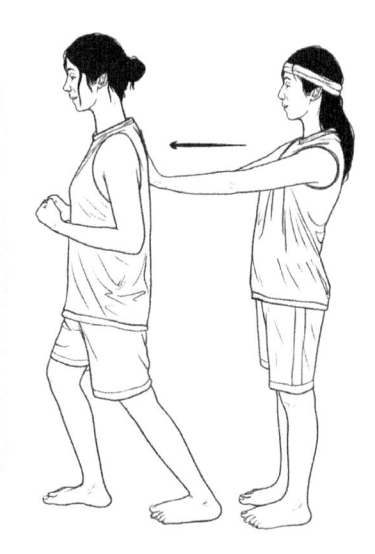

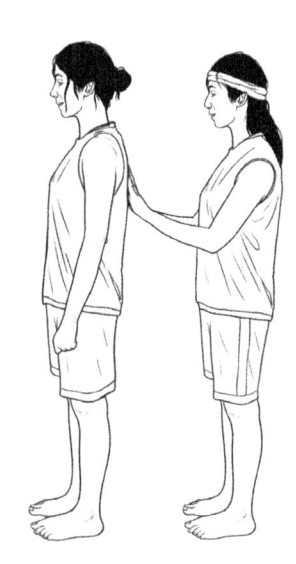

INSTRUCTIONS

1. Stand facing your partner, and place your right-hand palm on your partner's right-hand palm.
2. Take a step forward with your left leg to create a staggered stance, making sure that you are far enough for one of you to extend their arm while the other can stand back fully. You want to be able to push your partner's hand toward their chest.
3. Both of you push into each other to keep tension. The goal of the pushing movement is to make each other work for the movement. It's kind of like playing tug-of-war but with the pushing effect. However, you want to avoid resisting too hard; there should be a slow and steady movement between you.
4. Once you have mastered the tension, you need to bring your hand back toward your chest, and the other person should fully extend their arm. If you are starting with your hand toward your chest, push your partner's hand back as you extend your own. For the partner resisting, apply pressure as your hand is being moved.
5. Switch partners.

Repeat with your right arm for 8-12 pushes before changing sides.

EXERCISES YOU CAN DO WITH A PARTNER

PARTNER PULLS

INTRODUCTION

Like the partner pushes, the partner pull is a unilateral exercise to challenge your imbalances, while working on your back, bicep, and core muscles.

In this exercise, set up the same way as you did for the pushes, except this time you will grab your partner's hand like you are getting ready for an arm wrestle. Make sure you both create tension the entire time to work for the movement, but not so much that you or your partner can't move. As with partner pushes, the action between the partners should be smooth and fluid.

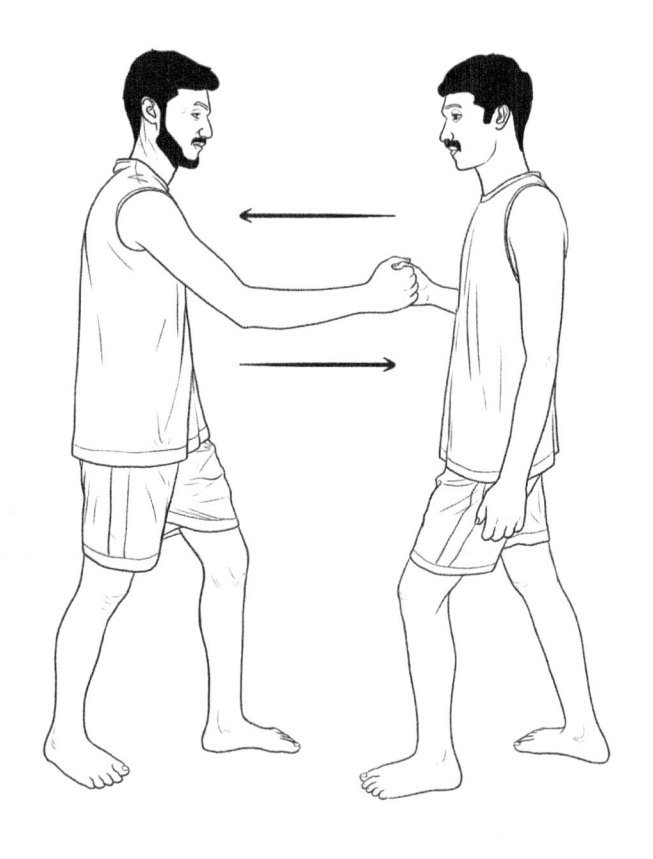

INSTRUCTIONS

1. Start by having one of your arms close to your chest, while the other has their arm extended.
2. Standing tall, the partner with the extended arm will pull their partner's hand towards them. The partner being pulled needs to add a little resistance to create the challenge.
3. Switch partners.

↻ Repeat with your right arm for 8-12 pushes before changing sides.

OTHER FUN ACTIVITIES TO DO WITH A PARTNER

Dancing

Dancing is not only a fun way to get low-impact cardio, but you also get the social aspect of it! For some older adults, it brings back good memories and experiences from their youth. Dancing is excellent to help prevent falls, improve your posture and flexibility, boost your energy and mood, and sharpen your mind. In addition, dancing creates a fun social atmosphere to engage with others.

If you are into ballroom dancing, waltzes are great for your heart health and breathing if you have a mild to a moderate heart condition. Participants who might have knee or hip discomfort from arthritis also found that their pain reduced significantly when they participated in a low-impact dance routine.

Playing Catch or Frisbee

Throwing a ball or a frisbee not only boosts your heart rate a little bit, but it also helps with your balance as you work to catch and throw the ball or frisbee! This activity is also a fun pastime for most, or something fun you can do with your grandkids.

CHAPTER TEN
EXERCISES WITH EQUIPMENT

You might find that you have your preferences when it comes to exercising. For example, some people prefer to use their body weight for strength training, or go for a walk or jog, all of which require no equipment. However, there are benefits to using equipment for your workouts, such as better control and resistance.

Our joints can quickly feel tired when they are overworked from high-intensity workouts. Equipment reduces the risk of injury by controlling the movement. Bodyweight is not always enough for resistance exercises, even for balance. This is why we use equipment. This allows our bodies to improve strength and balance with external forces like fitness equipment.

This chapter will focus on using medicine balls, resistance bands, dumbbells, and balance pads to get the most out of your workouts.

FIVE EXERCISE BALL EXERCISES

You will need a stability ball or a weighted medicine ball for the exercise ball exercises. For the weight recommendation for the medicine balls, you should use one between four and eight pounds.

Benefits of Medicine Balls

The use of a medicine (or weighted) ball dates back to ancient Greece, about 3,000 years ago! They used this form of exercise to help those healing from injuries as a recovery method. Today, medicine balls are popular in workout routines, because they can help improve your balance and core.

Each of these exercises is between a beginner and medium level.

EXERCISE BALL EXERCISES
TUMMY TWISTS

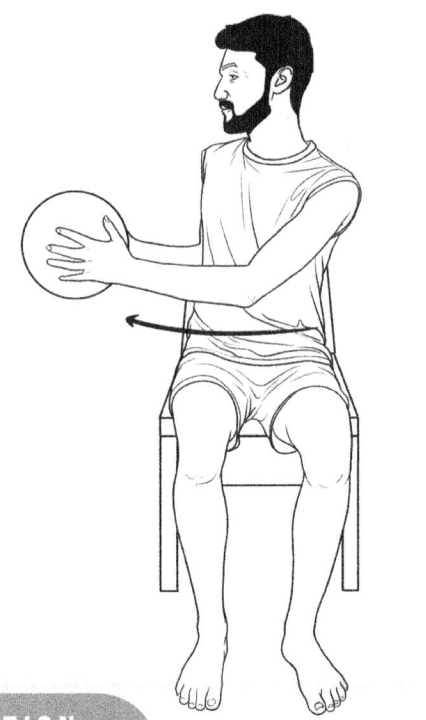

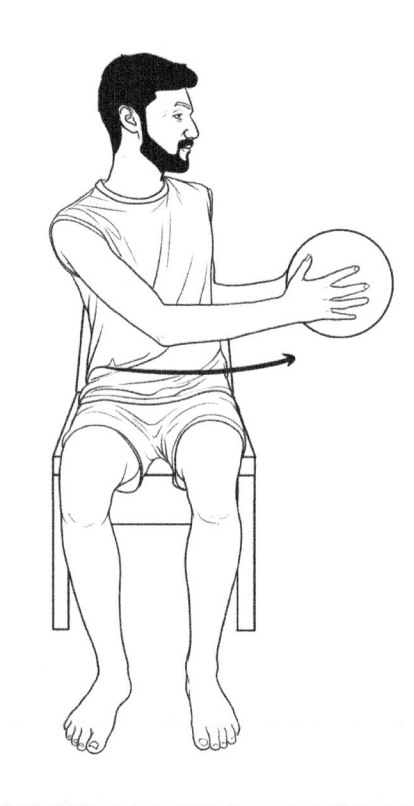

INTRODUCTION

Tummy Twists are great for your entire core, and can help stretch your spine. For this exercise, you will need a medicine ball or something similar to create the full tension in your abs. You will also need a chair.

INSTRUCTIONS

1. Sit comfortably in your chair toward the edge. You will need enough room in the back for the movement portion of this exercise.
2. Stick out your chest, and hold the medicine ball in front of you just a few inches above your lap. Your elbows should be slightly bent.
   Turn your upper body to the right while keeping the ball in front of you.
   Rotate towards your left in the same manner.
3. Finish by rotating to the middle to complete the full rotation.

Complete this exercise with 8-10 repetitions in two to three sets.

EXERCISE BALL EXERCISES
CIRCLE PRESS

INTRODUCTION

The circle press exercise helps to strengthen your chest and arm muscles. You will need a medicine ball and your chair for the exercise.

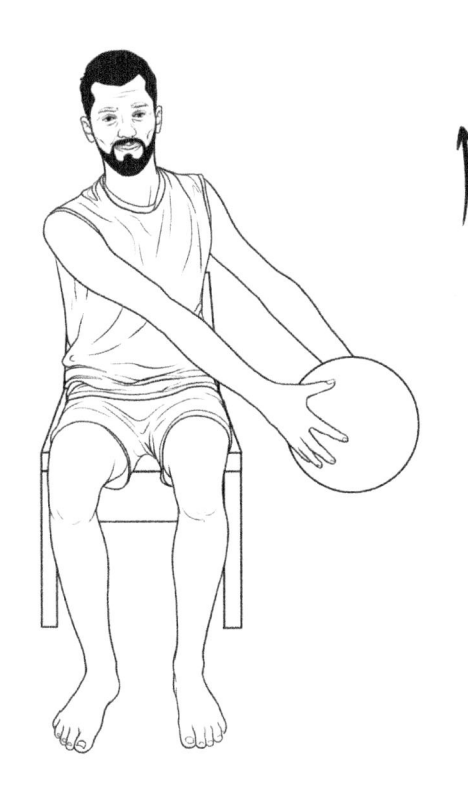

INSTRUCTIONS

1. Sit in your chair with your feet flat on the floor and facing forward. Be sure that your back is straight.
2. Engage and tighten your core muscles while you hold your medicine ball.
3. Bring the ball to chest height, keeping your elbows bent and forearms parallel to the floor.
4. Push your ball forward to straighten your arms. Hold for five seconds.
5. Bring the ball back while keeping your arms raised to complete one repetition. Repeat the movement.

↻ Complete two to three sets of this exercise with 8-12 reps. It is recommended to use a lighter-weighted medicine ball and, as you get stronger, increase the weight.

EXERCISE BALL EXERCISES
THIGH SQUEEZE

INTRODUCTION

This exercise helps to strengthen your inner thighs. You will need a medicine ball and a chair.

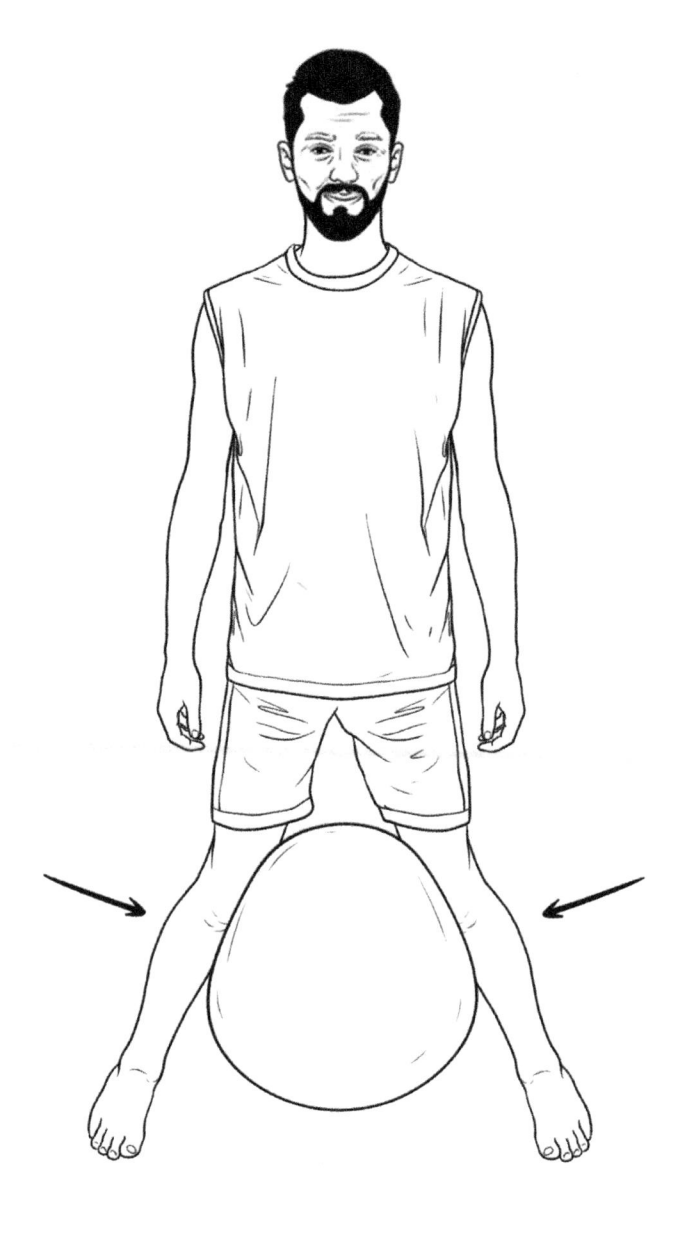

INSTRUCTIONS

1. Sit in your chair with your feet flat on the floor and facing forward. Be sure that your back is straight.
2. Place the medicine ball between your thighs.
3. Squeeze the ball and hold for 30 seconds, and then release.

Work to increase the time you can hold onto the ball. You will want to repeat this exercise until your inner thigh muscles feel fatigued.

EXERCISE BALL EXERCISES

SEATED BALL BALANCE

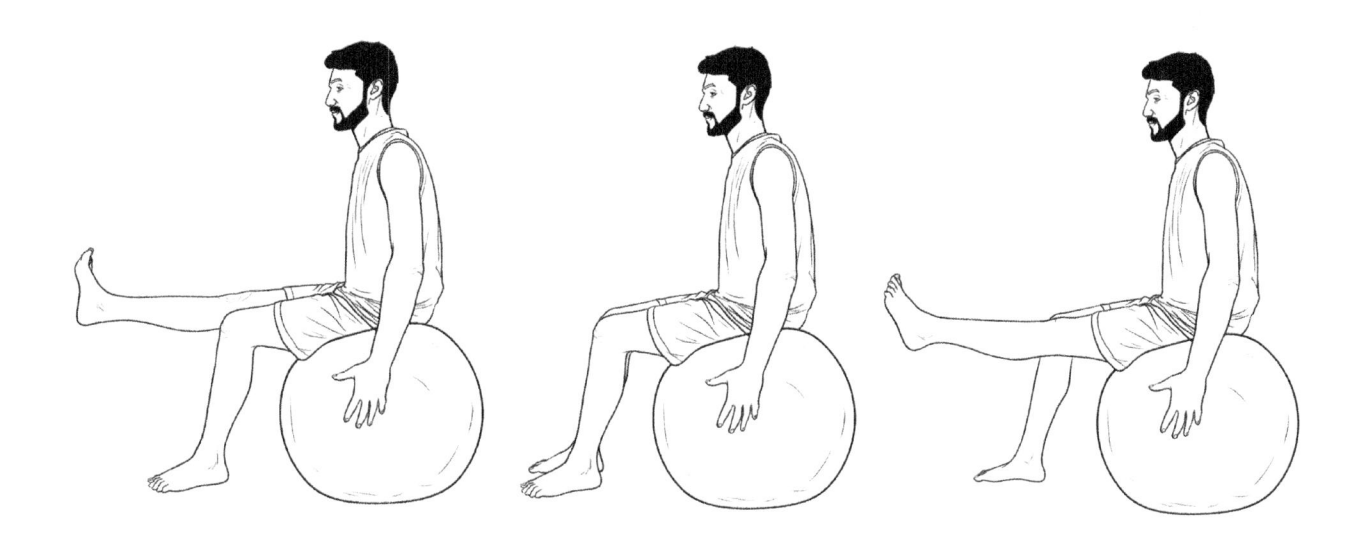

INTRODUCTION

The seated ball balance is one exercise that will challenge your balance while sitting on a stability ball. It is important that you are patient in perfecting this exercise. Try having a chair or a wall next to you for support if you need it, but the goal is to remain stable while seated on the stability ball.

INSTRUCTIONS

1. Sit on your stability ball with a straight spine.
2. Engage your abs to help you remain stable in the position.
3. Lift your right foot off of the floor a few inches.
4. Extend your leg as far as possible, and hold it in the air for five seconds.
5. Lower and repeat on the other side.

Repeat for 5-10 repetitions on each leg for two to three sets.

EXERCISE BALL EXERCISES
HIP LIFTS

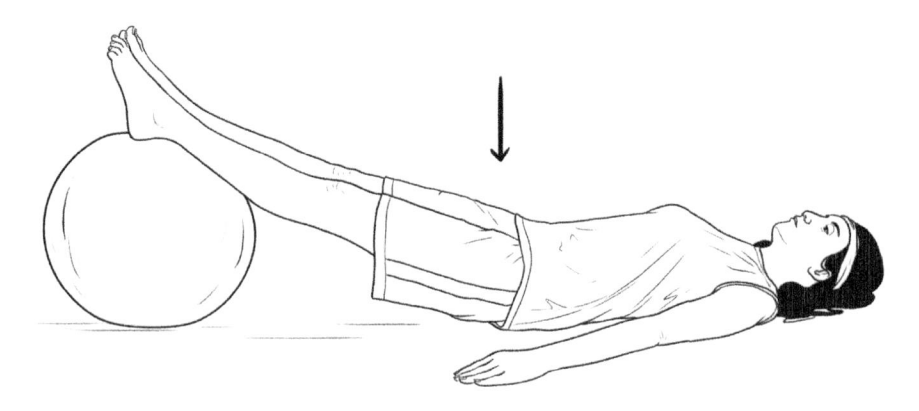

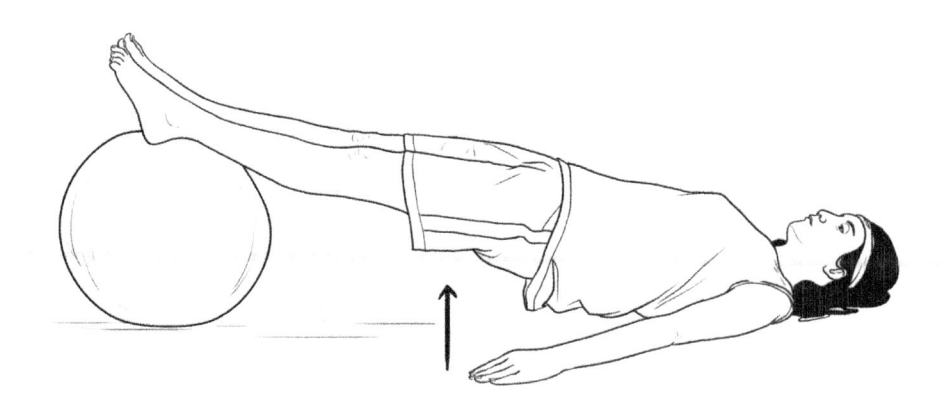

INTRODUCTION

Hip lifts help work on your balance by engaging your glutes and hamstrings. You will need your stability ball to perform the exercise.

INSTRUCTIONS

1. On the floor, lie down with your heels propped up on the stability ball. Engaging your abs, slowly lift your hips off the floor. Be sure to squeeze your glutes as you lift.
2. Stop until your body is in a straight diagonal line.
3. Hold for five seconds, then lower.

Repeat this movement 15 times.

FIVE RESISTANCE BAND EXERCISES

Using resistance bands in your workouts allows you to have versatile exercises that challenge you. In addition, studies have found that resistance bands have similar results in strength training as traditional equipment.

There are a few kinds of resistance bands you can use in your workout:
- Open-ended bands
- Resistance bands with handles
- Long loop resistance bands
- Lateral resistance bands

Benefits of Using Resistance Bands

Resistance bands in your workouts allow you to have various challenges. Though they are not weighted, they provide resistance in your exercises to challenge you. Here are some benefits that they can provide to you:

- Improve your flexibility
- Strengthen your muscles
- Help with imbalances
- Great for post-injury recovery
- Energize your brain's function

These five exercises are from a beginner to advanced level.

RESISTANCE BAND EXERCISES
EXTERNAL ROTATION

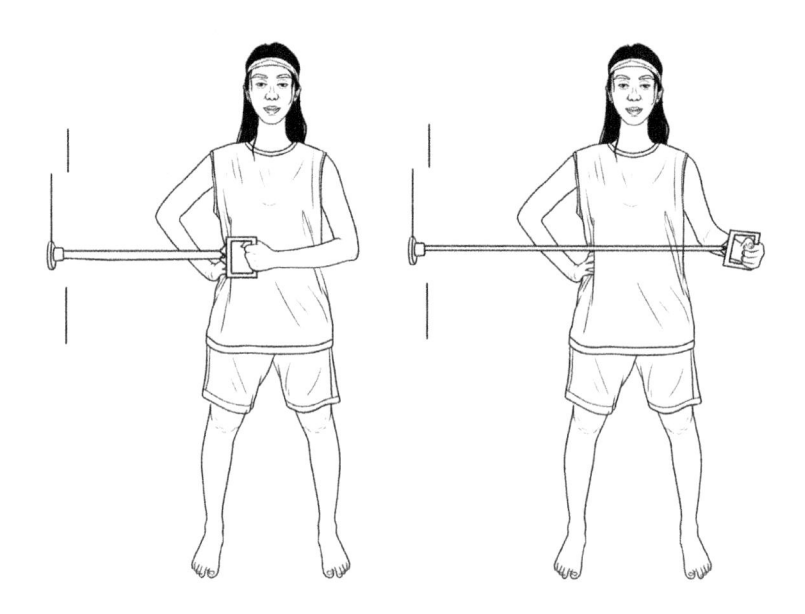

INTRODUCTION

The external rotation is designed to target your shoulder's rotator cuff. By strengthening your rotator cuff, you can lift your arms to reach those high-shelved items better. For this exercise, it's recommended to use a resistance band with handles.

INSTRUCTIONS

1. Hold the band's handle in your right hand with your knuckles facing.
   Hold the band about a foot from the handled end with your left hand to create tension.
2. Arms should be 90 degrees, with your left elbow pulled into your side.
   With your right hand, rotate your arm outwards, so your palm faces the front. Only rotate as far as is comfortable for you.
3. Release to rotate back into the starting position.
4. Switch sides after your last repetition.

Do the external rotation for 8-12 repetitions in two to three sets. One set completes a number of repetitions on each side.

RESISTANCE BAND EXERCISES
BENT OVER PULLDOWNS

INTRODUCTION

For the bent-over pulldowns, you will need a resistance band with handles. To set up, you will want to find a way to anchor your resistance band to your door frame. Door hooks usually come with resistance bands with handles.

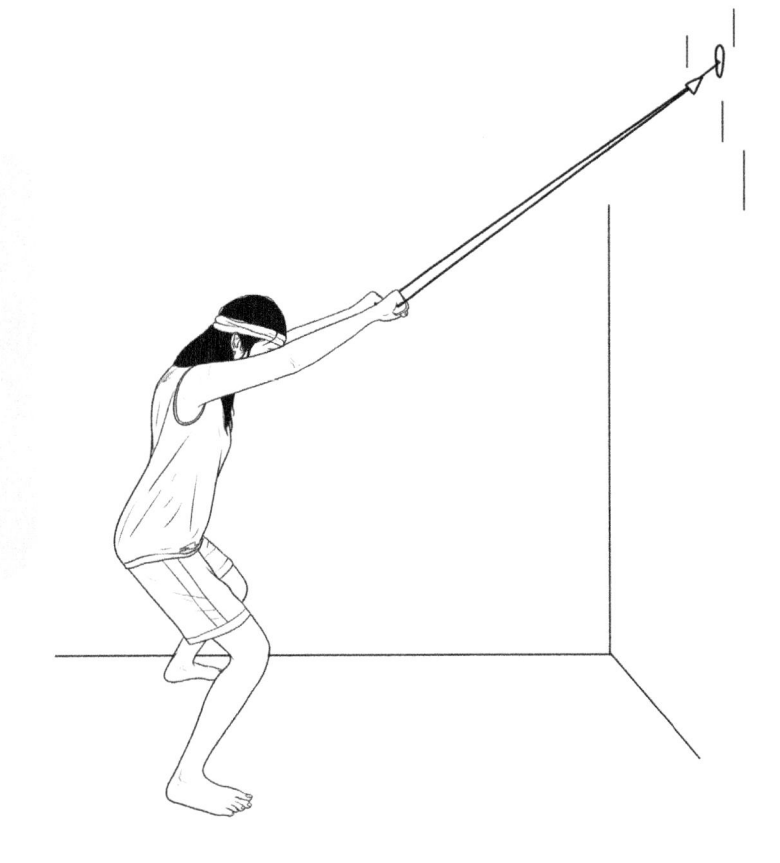

INSTRUCTIONS

1. Step back from the door to create tension in the band.
2. Stand with your feet slightly wider than your hips.
3. Grab the handles with your palms facing the door.
4. Bend at your hips, stopping at a 45-degree angle. Your arms should be straight out above you. If they are not, take a few more steps back until they are.
5. Tighten your core to support your back.
6. Pull the resistance band down, stopping when your hands are at your ears' level. You should feel your shoulder blades pulling down with the motion. Release to return to the start, and repeat.

Repeat the bent-over pulldown for 8-12 repetitions in two to three sets. One set completes a number of repetitions on each side.

RESISTANCE BAND EXERCISES
LEG EXTENSION

INTRODUCTION

This exercise requires a chair or a bench, and a long loop resistance band. The movement is going to target your quad muscles.

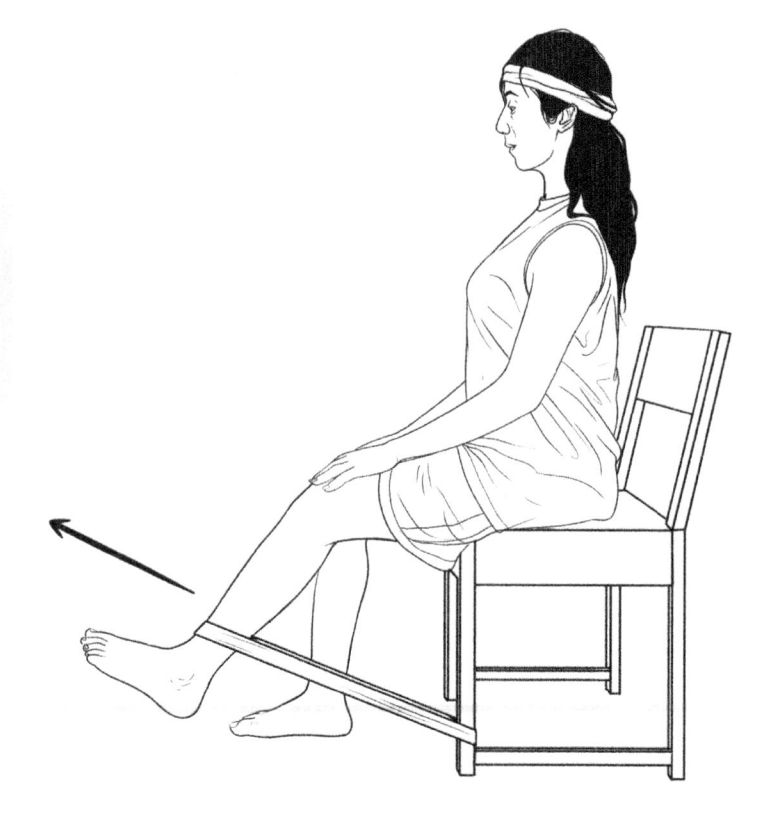

INSTRUCTIONS

1. Holding one end, anchor the long loop band in a low position on your chair or bench. If you are using a chair, it should be looping around the chair leg support.
2. Take the other end of the band and loop it around your right ankle. Position your feet hip-width apart.
3. Shift your weight to your supporting left leg as you elevate your right leg from the floor. Your ankle needs to be flexed, and your toes are facing the ceiling.
4. Extend your leg out until it is straight, or to what is comfortable for you. Slowly return to the start.

Complete 8-12 repetitions before switching to your left leg. Complete a total of two to three sets.

RESISTANCE BAND EXERCISES
STANDING ADDUCTION

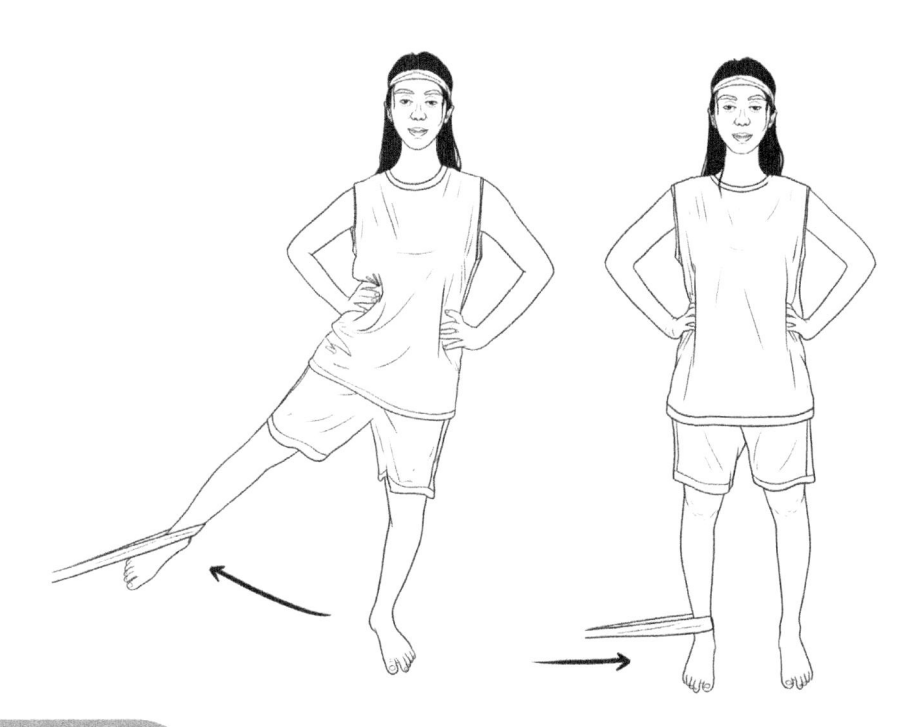

INTRODUCTION

This exercise is a great balancing challenge for you. You will need a lateral resistance band for this exercise.

INSTRUCTIONS

1. Place the lateral resistance band around your ankles.
2. Stand about hip-width apart to create tension in the band.
3. Shift your weight to your left leg.
4. Lift your right leg to the side, with your toes facing forward to activate your glutes.
5. Slowly lower your leg to the start.

Complete 8-12 repetitions before switching to your left leg. Complete a total of two to three sets.

Helpful tip: if you find balancing a challenge, use a chair or wall for support.

RESISTANCE BAND EXERCISES

LATERAL BAND WALK

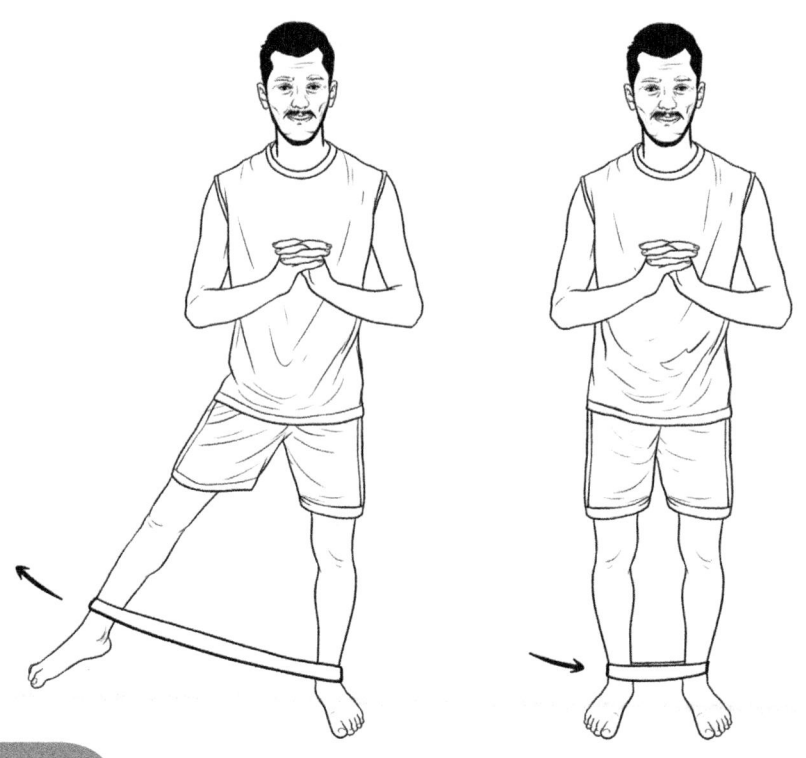

INTRODUCTION

The lateral band walk challenges your balance as you move sideways, something we don't do daily! Like the standing adduction, you will need the lateral resistance band, and the setup is the same, with the band around your ankle, and your legs shoulder-width apart. Again, you will need some space to move at least eight steps in each direction; a hallway might be your best space for this.

INSTRUCTIONS

1. Start in a half-squat position with your toes facing forward.
   Transfer your weight to your left leg, and begin stepping sideways with your right foot.
2. Once you have stepped eight times to the left, switch sides.

↻ Repeat this exercise in both directions 10 times.

FIVE DUMBBELL EXERCISES

It's a funny thought, but some people believe you somehow lose flexibility once you hit 50! However, as you have been learning throughout this book, you can continue to build and activate your muscles well past 50, and beyond.

Dumbbells are life-changing because they will help you stay in shape, regardless of age. Make sure to have three different dumbbell weights at your disposal. The weight increments you want to get are something in the lighter range (about five to eight pounds), medium range (10 to 12 pounds), and heavier range (about 15 to 17.5 pounds)

Benefits of Using Dumbells

Here are the benefits of incorporating dumbbells into your workout routine:
- Versatility to allow you to perform several movements, some of which can be done with the use of one dumbbell
- Correcting imbalances with the weight evenly distributed

Each of these exercises ranges between a beginner and medium level.

DUMBBELL EXERCISES
FRONT RAISE

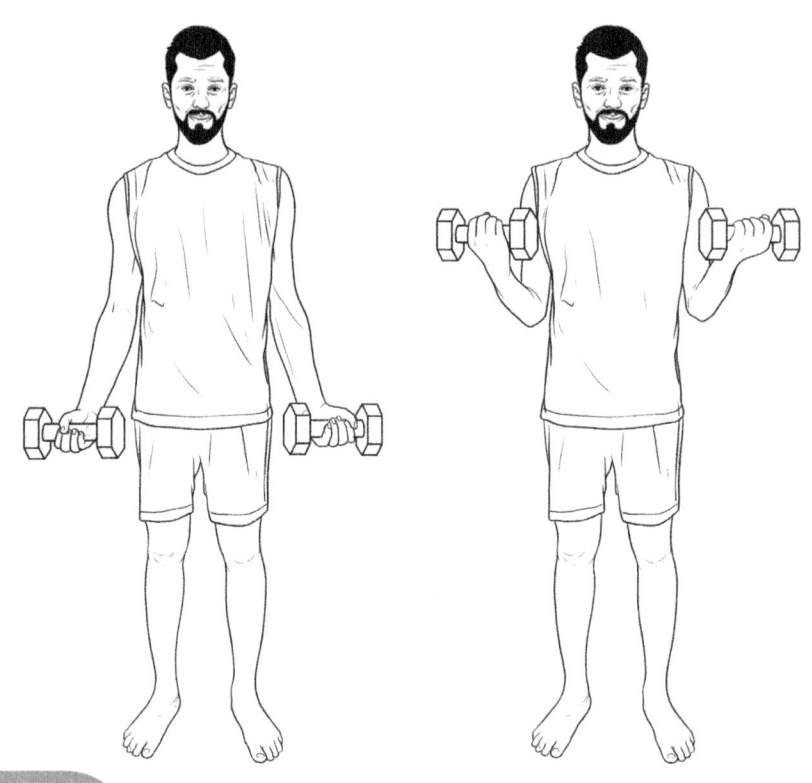

INTRODUCTION

The front raise is one of the most straightforward exercises you can do with a pair of dumbbells. It targets your shoulders from the front and side, chest muscles, and biceps. This exercise is a great way to strengthen your shoulder mobility.

Helpful tip: keep the movement smooth and controlled as you lift the weights. You will want to use lighter weights as well.

INSTRUCTIONS

1. Stand with a straight back and your legs hip distance apart and your hands in front of your thighs.
2. Exhale as you lift your dumbbells up to chest height. Inhale as you lower your dumbbells.

Repeat 8-12 times for two to three sets.

DUMBBELL EXERCISES
TRICEPS EXTENSIONS

INTRODUCTION

Triceps extensions are designed to strengthen the tricep muscles at the back of your upper arm. It is an isolated exercise, since the movement only involves your elbow. This exercise is best executed with a lighter weight to begin. You can increase your weight as you get stronger. It is recommended to use one dumbbell.

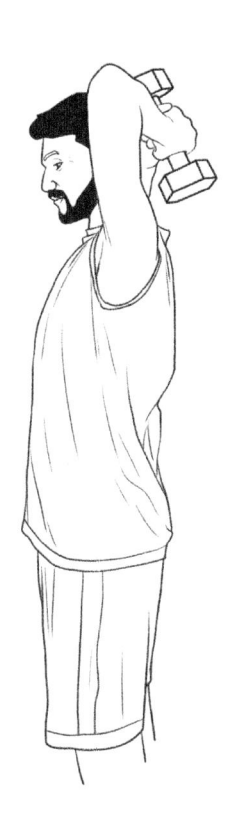

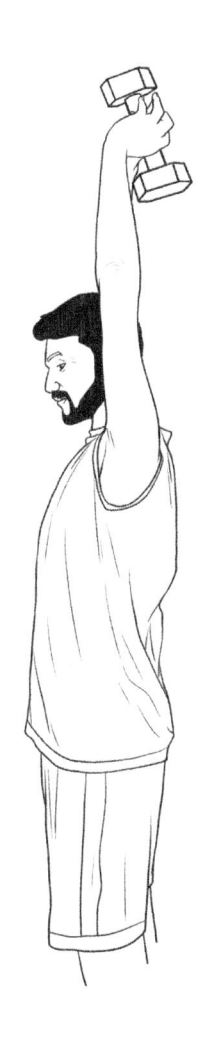

INSTRUCTIONS

1. To start your triceps extensions, stand with your feet in a staggered stance, with your right foot just slightly forward. Make sure to have your weight evenly distributed. Ensure your core is engaged in maintaining good posture.
2. Cup your dumbbell in both hands with your palms facing the ceiling.
3. Lift the weight over your head, and bring it behind your head. As you bend your elbows, ensure your elbows are hugging your head.
4. Extend both arms, and slowly lower the weight back behind your head, ensuring your neck remains neutral.

Repeat 8-12 times for two to three sets.

DUMBBELL EXERCISES

DUMBBELL LUNGE

INTRODUCTION

The dumbbell lunge involves a big step forward. Think of it as the forward version of the reverse lunges from chapter seven.

With weights in either hand, stand tall, and hang your arms at your sides. Your hands must be facing your thighs, and your feet be shoulder-width apart.

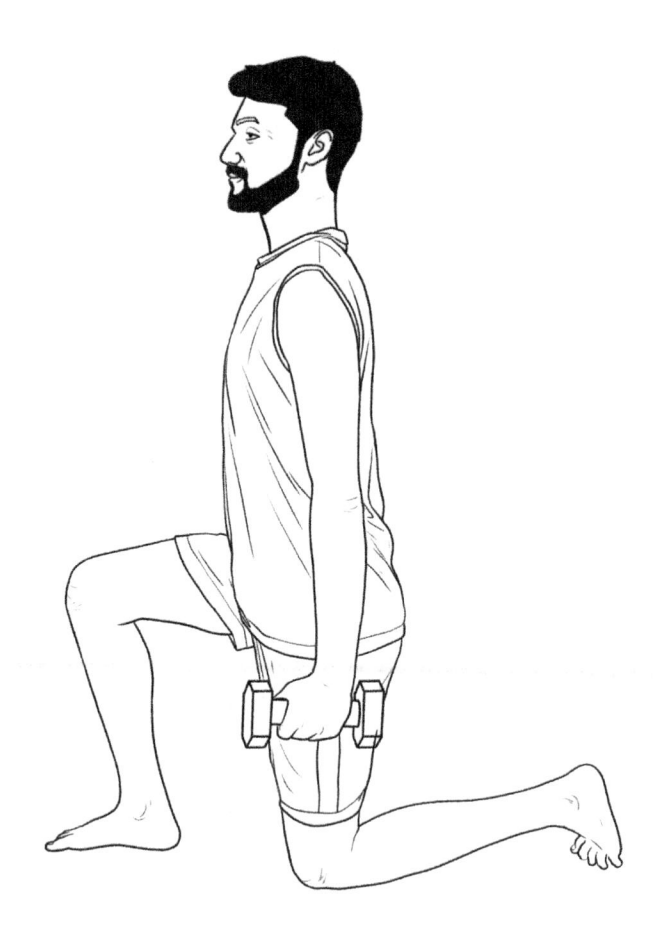

INSTRUCTIONS

1. As you inhale, take a step forward with your right leg to place your weight at your heel. Bend your knee as you land, until your quad is level with your hip.
2. Your left leg should be balanced on the toes, and bent.
3. Step back back into the starting position, and repeat the movement with your opposite leg.

On each leg repeat 8-12 times for two to three sets.

DUMBBELL EXERCISES
ONE LEGGED DEADLIFT

INTRODUCTION

Deadlifts are considered a compound weight exercise that has you pick a weight up from the floor by bending at your waist and hips, before returning to a standing position. The one-legged deadlift is a unilateral exercise to challenge your balance as you bend over with one leg lifting behind you. This exercise can be done using different tools.

For this exercise, you will only need one dumbbell.

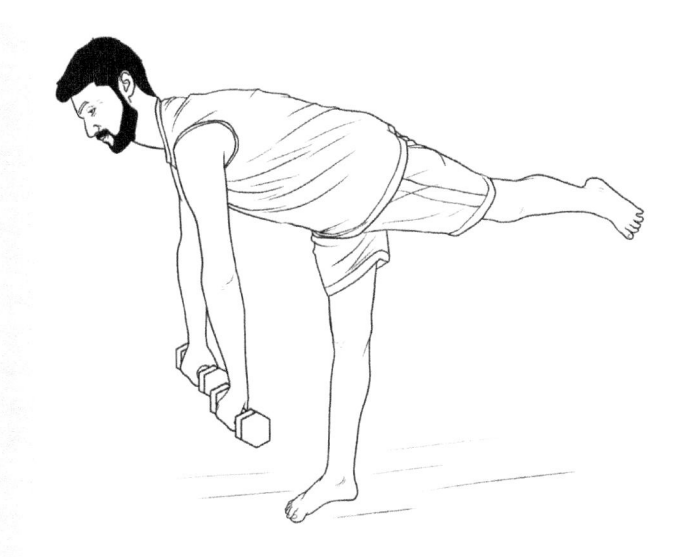

INSTRUCTIONS

1. Start with your dumbbell in your left hand.
2. Stand with your legs hip-width apart with your feet under your hips. Make sure to keep your knees soft. Your dumbbell should be in front of your thigh with your palm.
3. Push the weight down to your right foot as you shift your weight over.
4. Begin to bring your left foot up behind you as you bend over. Ensure you are hinging at your hips to tip your torso forward. Your torso should be nearly parallel to the floor, and your arms straight.
5. Once you reach the bottom position, begin bringing your left foot back to tip your torso back to the starting position.

↻ Repeat on each leg 8-12 times for two to three sets.
   Helpful tip: if you find your balance hard to keep, use a chair or wall for support.

DUMBBELL EXERCISES
ROMANIAN LUNGE

INTRODUCTION

The Romanian lunge, also known as the Bulgarian lunge, is a version of a single-leg squat. Your back leg will be elevated on a chair to challenge your balance. You can use one moderate-heavy dumbbell or two lighter dumbbells in front of your stomach.

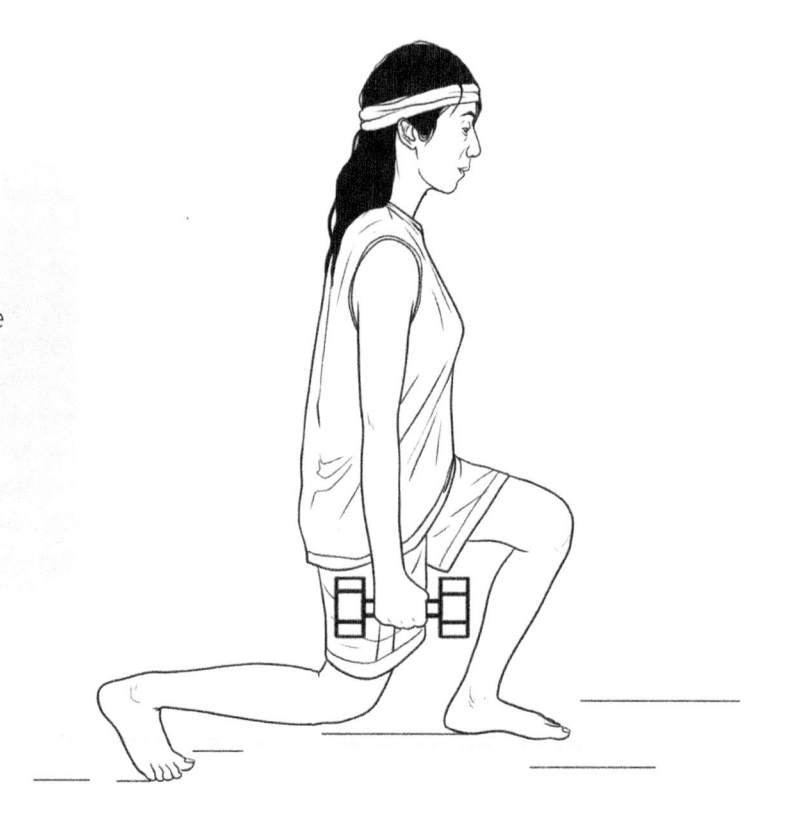

INSTRUCTIONS

1. Stand about two feet in front of your chair with your legs hip-width apart. Ensure to engage your core, bring your shoulders back, and your chest broad.

2. Lift your right foot and place it on the chair behind you. There are two ways you can rest your foot on the chair. The first being to identify the top of your foot on your chair, with your ankle joint aligned to the edge. Your other option is to flex your ankle, and use the ball of your foot and toes to find your balance, similar to a regular lunge exercise. Your elevated back foot's job is to help you remain balanced while you turn your awareness to your working leg.

3. As you engage your core, begin to bend your left knee. Let your supporting knee and ankle bend naturally as you bend downwards, but make sure not to put the load on your back leg.

4. Keeping the weight load natural, press through your heel to return to the start.

↻ Repeat on each leg 8-12 times for two to three sets.

FIVE BALANCE PAD EXERCISES

Having to depend on someone to keep you stable on your feet, or feeling the fear of falling and injuring yourself, is not fun. Balance pad exercises are an excellent way to maintain your overall balance.

You can do them with a friend, or on your own at home. When trying out these exercises, make sure you have something nearby to support you if needed.

Benefits of Using Balance Pads

Balance pad exercises allow you to engage your smaller muscles with the bigger ones. For example, standing on a balance pad alone can help strengthen the smaller muscles around your ankle, while working out your core and feet muscles. You'll also find stability in your knees, ankles, hips, and shoulders joints, and minimize the risk of injuries. For older adults, balance can help you prevent falls.

BALANCE PAD EXERCISES
SIDE-TO-SIDE STEPS

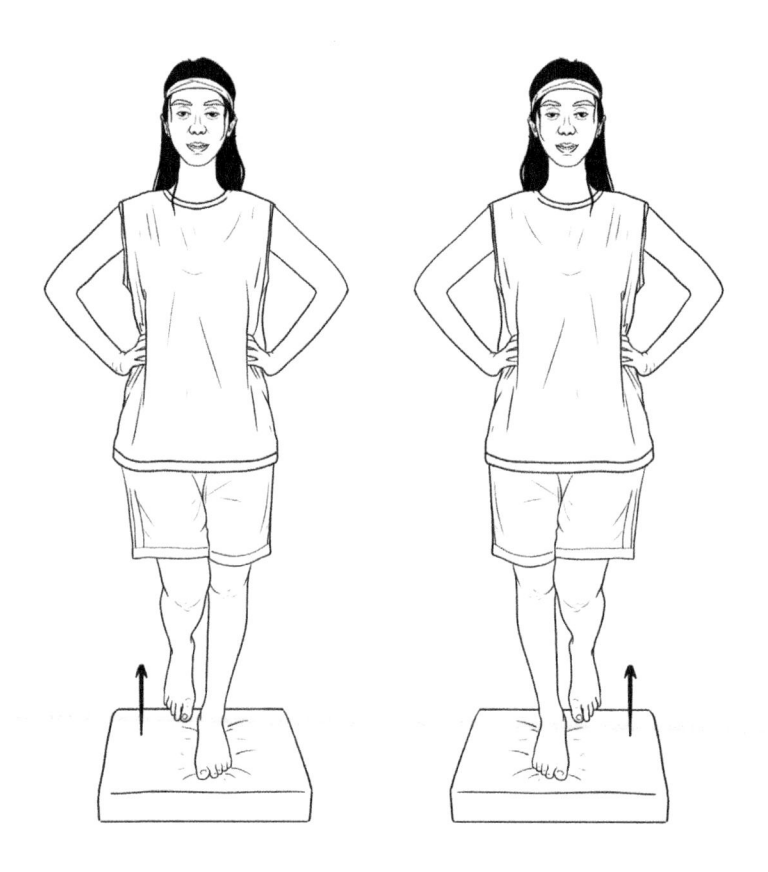

INSTRUCTIONS

1. Begin the side-to-side steps by standing on your balance pad with your feet. Transfer your weight to your right foot, while slowly lifting your left foot from the pad.
2. Hold the stance for five seconds, then put your left foot down. Lift your right foot right away.

Repeat the exercise 5-10 times on each side.

BALANCE PAD EXERCISES

MARCHING IN PLACE

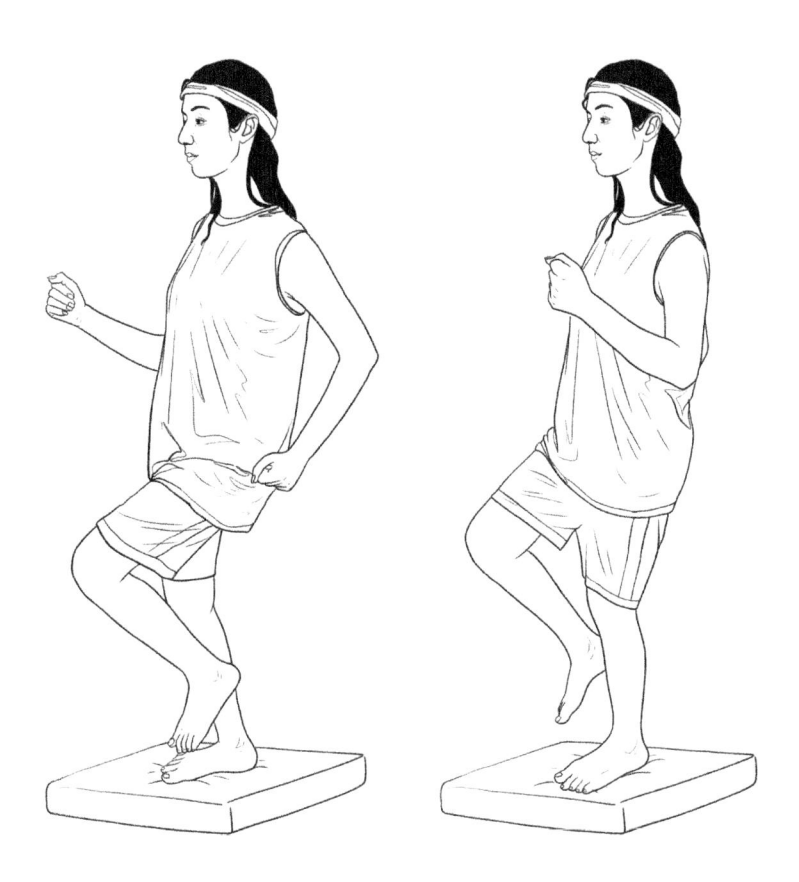

INSTRUCTIONS

1. Begin standing on your balance pad like you did your side-to-side steps.
2. Start marching on your balance pad, bringing one leg up at a time as high as possible. Move your arms simultaneously (as you did during Chapter six's marching on the spot exercise).

- Continue for 30 to 60 seconds; you can play some music too.

BALANCE PAD EXERCISES

SINGLE LEG BALANCE

INSTRUCTIONS

1. Stand on your balance pad with your feet close together.
2. Bring your arms to the side for balance (as if you were walking a tightrope).
3. Bring your knee up as far as you can. Try to have your knee to hip level if you can.
4. Hold for 20 seconds, and lower your leg to the pad. Switch legs.

↻ Repeat 5-10 times on each side.

BALANCE PAD EXERCISES
SQUATS

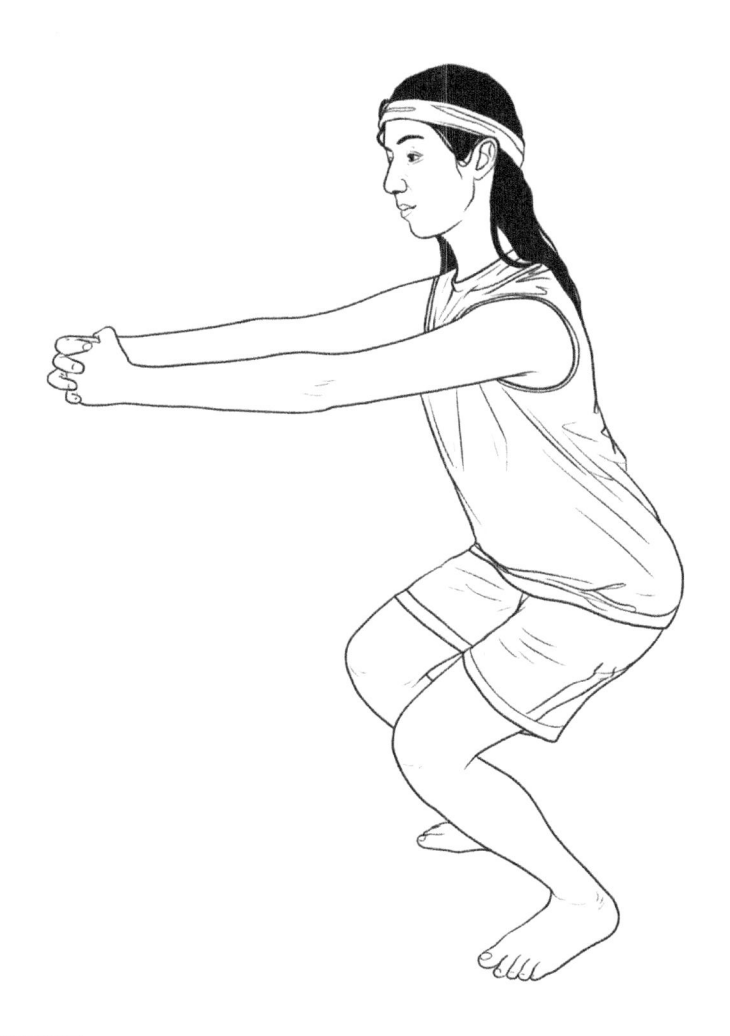

INSTRUCTIONS

1. Stand on your balance pad with your legs hip-width apart.
2. Bring your arms out in front of you.
3. As you have done in your squats, slowly bend your knees, keeping them behind your toes.
4. Lower as far as you can, then return to the beginning position.

Repeat 8-12 times.

BALANCE PAD EXERCISES

FRONT ELEVATED LUNGE

INTRODUCTION

The front elevated lunge—with your front leg elevated on your balance pad—will challenge your balance.

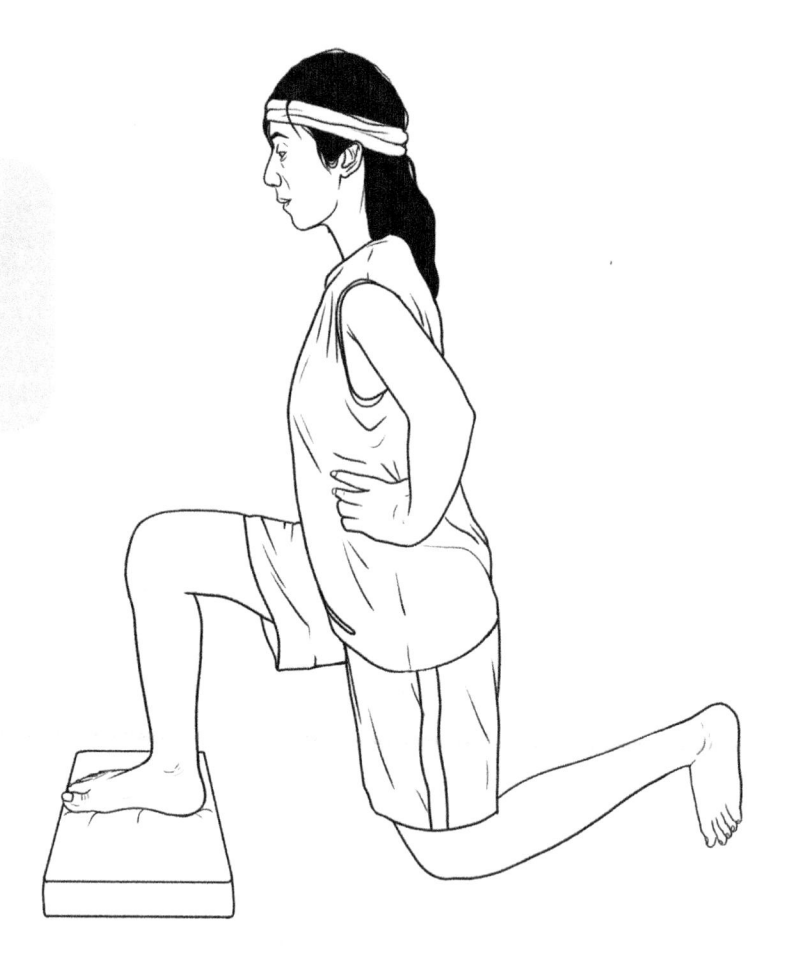

INSTRUCTIONS

1. Place your right foot on your balance pad, and your left leg about a foot behind you. Make sure your staggered stance is even.
2. Bend your front and back leg to 90 degrees, or as comfortable as it is for you. Stand back up and repeat.

↻ Repeat 5-10 times on each side.

CHAPTER ELEVEN
WEEKLY WORKOUT PLANNER

This chapter provides a guideline of workouts that you can try. When choosing your workout plan, decide what you want the most out of your training. For example, do you want to improve your upper body strength? Or, maybe you want to improve your range of motion in your lower body?

The first three workout plans are also based on your fitness level. Of course, these are just guidelines, and you can always mix it up based on your needs.

WORKOUT PLANS YOU CAN FOLLOW

The beginning, medium, and advanced levels will take about 30 minutes. However, closer to the end of this chapter, you'll find some that you can fit into a 10-minute block of time.

These workout plans also have a morning and night routine you can follow daily, to continue supporting your flexibility and posture.

Beginner Level Workout Plan

Monday

- 5-10 Head Rotations
- 5-10 Shoulder Rolls
- Three to five Seated Overhead Stretch
- 8-12 Tricep Extensions (do two to three sets)
- 8-12 Bicep Curls (do two to three sets)
- 8-12 Front Raise (do two to three sets)

Tuesday

- 5-10 Single Leg Stance (hold for 10 seconds)
- 5-10 Single Leg Raise (hold for 10 seconds)
- Three one minute Marching on the Spot
- Three one minute Side-to-Side Taps
- Three one minute Lateral Step
- Three one minute Heel Touches

Wednesday

- 5-10 Head Rotations
- 5-10 Shoulder Rolls
- Three to five Neck Stretches (hold for 15 to 20 seconds on each side)
- Three to five Lower Back Stretches (hold for 15 to 20 seconds)
- Three to five Hip Stretches (hold 15 to 20 seconds on each side)
- Three to five Quadricep Stretches (hold for 15 to 20 seconds on each side)

Thursday

For these exercises, you will do them at last three to five times, unless otherwise noted.

- Seated Backbends (hold for 20 seconds)
- Hip Stretch (hold for 10 to 20 seconds on each side)
- Eight Seated Half-Rollbacks (hold for 30 seconds)
- Seated Forward Roll-Ups (do two to three sets)
- 8-12 Side Bends (do two to three sets)
- 8-12 Tummy Twists (do two to three sets)

Friday

- Two to three Calf Stretches on each leg (hold for 20 seconds)
- Three to five Quadricep Stretches (hold for 15 to 20 seconds on each side)
- Three one minute Marching on the Spot
- 8-12 Hip Extensions (do two to three sets)
- 8-12 Lunges (do two to three sets)
- 8-12 Leg Extension (do two to three sets)

Saturday

Rest day! Find a friend and go for a walk, play catch, or toss a frisbee. Do something relaxing that won't strain your muscles.

Sunday

- Ladder (repeating 5-10 times)
- Three one minute Side-to-Side Taps
- Three one minute Heel-to-Toe Touches
- 10 Side-to-Side Steps on each side (do two to three sets)
- 10 Toe Lifts (hold for 10 seconds each)

Medium Level Workout Plan

Monday

- Three to five Seated Side Stretches (hold for 10 seconds on each side)
- 5-10 Balancing Wands on each side
- 5-10 Leg Raises (hold for 10 seconds on each raise)
- 10 Rock the Boats (do two to three sets)
- Three minutes of Stepping Stones
- 8-12 Knee Ups (do two to three sets)

Tuesday

- One minute of Tree Pose on each side
- Thigh Squeezes, holding the medicine ball for 30 seconds each
- 8-12 Reverse Lunges (do two to three sets)
- 8-12 Modified Squats (do two to three sets)
- 8-12 Standing Adductions (do two to three sets)
- Single Leg Crossbody three times on each side

Wednesday

- Five Heel-to-Toe Walking (going forward and back counts as one)
- 15 to 20 Step Ups
- 5-10 Single Leg Balance (hold for 20 seconds)

- 5-10 Seated Ball Balance (do two to three sets)
- Obstacles
- Zig-Zag Walking

Thursday

- Two to three Modified Planks (hold for at least 30 seconds each)
- 8-10 Supermans
- 8-12 Diagonal Outward Shoulder Raises (do two to three sets)
- 8-12 Bent Over Pulldowns (do two to three sets)

Friday

For this group of exercises, you will hold the stretch for 15 to 20 seconds three to five times, unless otherwise noted.

- Neck Stretches
- Seated Side Stretches (hold for 10 seconds on each side)
- Shoulder and Upper Arm Stretches
- Lower Back Stretches
- Two to three Calf Stretches on each leg
- Quadricep Stretches

Saturday

For each of these exercises, you will do two to three sets with 8-12 repetitions.

- Tricep Kickbacks
- Circle Press
- Diagonal Outward Shoulder Raises
- Diagonal Inward Shoulder Raises
- Overhead Press

Sunday

Rest day.

Advanced Level Workout Plan

Monday

For each of these exercises, you will do two to three sets with 8-12 repetitions, unless otherwise noted.

- Knee Extensions
- Heel Slides
- Extended Leg Raises
- Leg Kicks
- Fifteen Hip Lifts

Tuesday

For each of these exercises, you will do two to three sets with 8-12 repetitions, unless otherwise noted.

- External Rotations
- Bent Over Pulldowns
- Leg Extension
- Standing Adduction
- 10 Lateral Band Walks in each direction 10 times

Wednesday

For each of these exercises, you will do them three times at one minute intervals, unless otherwise noted.

- 8-12 Knee Ups (do two to three sets)
- Three Step-ups at a Faster Pace
- Three Heel-to-Toe Touches
- Lateral Steps
- Aerobic Challenge two times

Thursday

Rest day.

Friday

For each of these exercises, you will do two to three sets with 8-12 repetitions, unless otherwise noted.

- 10-15 Sit-to-Stand
- Leg Extensions
- Front Elevated Lunge
- Reverse Lunge
- One Legged Deadlift
- Romanian Deadlift

Saturday

For each of these exercises, you will do them three to five times in 10 to 20 second intervals each, unless otherwise noted.

- Neck Stretch
- 10 Upper Body Rotations (five in each direction)
- Seated Side Stretch
- Hip Stretch
- Seated Backbend
- Quadriceps Stretch

Sunday

For this list of exercises, you will need your balance pad. Each exercise will be done 5-10 times, unless otherwise noted.

- Side-to-Side Steps
- Marching in place for 30 to 60 seconds, five times
- Single Leg Balance

- 8-12 Squats (two to three sets)
- Front Elevated Lunges

Stretching Morning and Night Routines

Stretching is one of the greatest things you can do for your body to keep it flexible and reduce pain. Doing some stretching after you wake up and prior to going to bed will help you manage your pain throughout the day, and as you sleep.

Repeat three to five times for each of these stretches while holding between 10 and 20 seconds each.

Monday to Sunday Mornings

- Neck Stretch
- Seated Backbend
- Seated Overhead Stretch
- Shoulder Rolls
- Seated Hip Stretch

Monday to Sunday Evenings

- Neck Stretch
- Calf Stretch
- Shoulder and Upper Arm Stretch
- Quadriceps Stretch
- Lower Back Stretch
- Hip Stretch

Ten Minute Routines

Ten minute routines are an excellent, quick way to boost your heartrate, and get a little more activity into your day. You can do this in between commercial breaks, or while you are cooking a meal.

Do each of these seven times at 60 second intervals, with a 30 second rest. Each day you will alternate on the set of exercises.

Monday, Wednesday, and Friday
- Marching on the spot
- Step ups
- Toe Lifts

Tuesday, Thursday, Saturday
- Lateral steps
- Heel-to-toe touches
- Knee ups

Sunday
Rest day

Thank You!

This is a quick message of thanks that you picked my book from dozens of other books available for you to purchase.

Thank you for getting this and reading this all the way to the end.

Before you go, I'd like to ask a minute of your time to leave me a review on Amazon. As an indie author, every review (or star rating) matters as it helps our books become more visible on the platform thus in turn helps us reach and help more people.

Here are the links for your convenience:

Leave a review in:

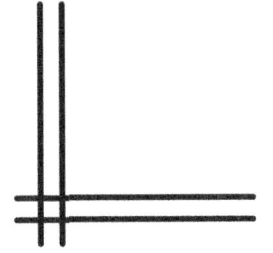

| US | UK | CA |

CONCLUSION

As you read this book, you learned different exercises that you can implement in your workout, to strengthen and improve your balance. Among the different techniques you learned, you also learned what causes imbalances and how to correct them.

- Why being balanced is beneficial to you
- The science behind imbalance issues
- General tips to finding your balance
- Warm-up exercises to challenge your balance
- How to focus on specific muscle groups
- Challenging your vestibular organ
- Activities you can do with a workout buddy
- Exercising with equipment and the benefits they can provide to you

There is much more you can do outside of this guidance, and this merely serves as a framework. Various facilities offer programs that can help to improve your balance. These include water aerobics, water Zumba, or senior-friendly pilates.

All the wisdom imparted by this book has equipped you to be knowledgeable about the exercises you can do for balance and strength as a senior. We strongly encourage you to stay dedicated to one of the plans mentioned in this book, to help you get your muscles moving, and your balance improving.

As you exercise and do some training, you will see that your fitness is but a foundation that you can add onto, regardless of the pace it takes to get you there.

GLOSSARY

Adductor Magnus: This triangular muscle extends over the entire medial side of the thigh.

Cortisol: The main stress hormone, cortisol is responsible for how we react to fight-or-flight situations. Cortisol also helps to increase glucose in the bloodstream, and increase your brain's use of glucose and other substances to help repair tissues.

Dumbbell: A short bar with weights on either end.

Endorphins: Any of a group of hormones discharged inside the brain and nervous system, to activate the body's opiate receptors, such as pain relief.

Glucose: The simple sugar which provides energy.

Gluteus: The large muscles in the buttocks.

Lumbar: Contains five bones in your lower back.

Lumbopelvic: How the lumbar spine moves in combination with the pelvis.

Lymphocytes: A smaller form of the white blood cell.

Medial: Toward the middle or center.

Osteoarthritis A condition of arthritis that affects joints when degenerative changes happen in the cartilage.

Phagocytes: A cell within the body capable of devouring microorganisms and dead tissue cells.

Proprioception: The ability to sense movement, action, and location.

Rung: The crosspiece between a ladder's frame.

Tandem: Having two things arranged in front or behind one another.

REFERENCES

7 Balance Pad Exercises for Seniors. (2018, May 1). ProsourceFit. https://www.prosourcefit.com/blogs/news/7-balance-pad-exercises-for-seniors

8 ways dancing boosts your physical and mental health. (2019). Chartwell.com. https://chartwell.com/en/blog/2019/07/8-ways-dancing-boosts-your-physical-and-mental-health

12 Best Elderly Balance Exercises For Seniors to Reduce the Risk of Falls. (2019). Eldergym® Senior Fitness. https://eldergym.com/elderly-balance/

21 Chair Exercises for Seniors: Complete Visual Guide - California Mobility. (2018, December 14). California Mobility. https://californiamobility.com/21-chair-exercises-for-seniors-visual-guide/

Acosta, K. (2021, August 2). A Guide To The Best Exercises For Seniors. Forbes Health. https://www.forbes.com/health/healthy-aging/best-exercises-for-seniors/

Ambrose, A. F., Paul, G., & Hausdorff, J. M. (2013). Risk factors for falls among older adults: A review of the literature. Maturitas, 75(1), 51–61. https://doi.org/10.1016/j.maturitas.2013.02.009

American Heart Association. (2014). Warm Up, Cool Down. Www.heart.org. https://www.heart.org/en/healthy-living/fitness/fitness-basics/warm-up-cool-down

Baiera, V. (2021, June 21). 25 Fun Balance Exercises for the Elderly. Step2Health. https://step2health.com/blogs/news/25-fun-balance-exercises-for-the-elderly

Balance Pad: Exercises for Your Workout | Technogym. (2021, October 12). Technogym - Gym Equipment and Fitness Solutions for Home and Business. https://www.technogym.com/us/newsroom/balance-pad-exercises-workout

Basic Facts about Balance Problems | Aging & Health A-Z | American Geriatrics Society | HealthInAging.org. (2016). Healthinaging.org. https://www.healthinaging.org/a-z-topic/balance-problems/basic-facts

Bedosky, L. (2021, March 13). The Best Core Exercises for Seniors. Get Healthy U | Chris Freytag. https://gethealthyu.com/best-core-exercises-for-seniors/

Brown, N. (2019, April 26). The Top 5 Benefits Of Using Medicine Balls In Your Workouts - The Home Gym. The Home Gym. https://the-home-gym.com/the-top-5-benefits-of-using-medicine-balls-in-your-workouts

Bubnis, D. (2019, October 31). How to Do Front Dumbbell Raises: Instructions and More. Healthline. https://www.healthline.com/health/exercise-fitness/front-dumbbell-raise

Bubnis, D. (2021, May 7). Deadlift Benefits: 8 Ways This Exercise Supercharges Results. Healthline. https://healthline.com/health/fitness/deadlift-benefits

Bucci, R. (2020, July 8). The Importance of Warming Up. Www.resultspt.com. https://www.resultspt.com/blog/posts/the-importance-of-warming-up

Centers for Disease Control and Prevention. (2019). How much physical activity do older adults need? Cdc.gov. https://www.cdc.gov/physicalactivity/basics/older_adults/index.htm

Cordier, A. (2018, February 9). 5 Reasons Why Warm Up Exercises Are Important -. Fitathletic.com. https://fitathletic.com/5-reasons-warm-exercises-important/

Cronkleton, E. (2020, July 28). Never Skip a Leg Day: Benefits, Cautions, and More. Healthline. https://www.healthline.com/health/exercise-fitness/never-skip-leg-day#benefits-of-leg-days

Davis, K. (2015, February 13). 33 Resistance Band Exercises You Can Do Literally Anywhere. Greatist; Healthline Media. https://greatist.com/fitness/resistance-band-exercises

Evans, L. (2018, February 12). Why are hip exercises so important? Bare Biology. https://www.barebiology.com/blogs/news/why-are-hip-exercises-so-important

Exercise safety | betterhealth.vic.gov.au. (n.d.). Www.betterhealth.vic.gov.au. https://www.betterhealth.vic.gov.au/health/healthyliving/exercise-safety#exercise-safety-advice

Exercising with Chronic Conditions. (n.d.). National Institute on Aging. https://www.nia.nih.gov/health/exercising-chronic-conditions

Export, J. (2017, May 29). 7 Health Benefits of Plank Exercises (+5 Plank Variations You Should Know). HealthCorps. https://www.healthcorps.org/fitness-2017-05-plankexercises/

Fancy, L. (2020, March 20). 6 Ways for Seniors to Stay Safe While Exercising. Home Care Assistance Winnipeg, Manitoba. https://www.homecareassistancewinnipeg.ca/how-can-aging-adults-exercise-safely/

Fay, R. R., Popper, A. N., Highstein, S. M., & Lovett, G. (2004). Vestibular System. Springer.

Finn, A. (2021, November 28). Walking Exercises to Build Strength While You Stroll. Well+Good. https://www.wellandgood.com/walking-exercises/

Freutal, N. (2016, January 13). Stretching Exercises for Seniors: Improve Mobility. Healthline. https://www.healthline.com/health/senior-health/stretching-exercises

Frey, M. (2022, July 28). How to Do a Triceps Extension. Verywell Fit. https://www.verywellfit.com/how-to-do-a-triceps-extension-techniques-benefits-variations-5082227

Got Back Pain? How the Superman Exercise Can Help. (2021, May 10). Cleveland Clinic. https://health.clevelandclinic.org/got-back-pain-how-the-superman-exercise-can-help/

Goulding, P. (2019, June 25). Isolation versus compound exercises | Nuffield Health. Www.nuffieldhealth.com. https://www.nuffieldhealth.com/article/isolation-versus-compound-exercises

Hain, T. (n.d.). Home-Based Dizziness Exercises. VeDA. https://vestibular.org/article/diagnosis-treatment/treatments/home-based-exercise/

Hand Eye Coordination: Tips for Improvement. (2016, November 16). Healthline. https://www.healthline.com/health/hand-eye-coordination#aging

Health, M. of. (n.d.). What Contributes to Falls? - Province of British Columbia. Www2.Gov.bc.ca. https://www2.gov.bc.ca/gov/content/family-social-supports/seniors/health-safety/disease-and-injury-care-and-prevention/fall-prevention/what-contributes-to-falls#:~:text=Biological%20risk%20factors%20include%20 advanced

Hegg, J. (2018, May 2). 4 Great Reasons to Find a Workout Partner After 60. Sixty and Me. https://sixtyandme.com/4-great-reasons-to-find-a-workout-partner-after-60/

Hildreth, D. (2021, October 25). 11 Irresistible Benefits of Resistance Bands. Greatist. https://greatist.com/fitness/benefits-of-resistance-bands

Ishler, J. (2021, June 17). Could Your Hips Hold the Key to Your Emotions? Some Experts Say Yes. Healthline. https://www.healthline.com/health/mind-body/the-powerful-connection-between-your-hips-and-your-emotions

Kashouty, R. (2021, November 5). The Vestibular System: What It is and How It Affects Balance. Premier Neurology & Wellness Center. https://premierneurologycenter.com/blog/the-vestibular-system-what-it-is-and-how-it-affects-balance/

Kutcher, M. (2019, October 6). Best Leg Strengthening Exercises For Seniors | Seniors Fitness. More Life Health - Seniors Health & Fitness. https://morelifehealth.com/articles/the-10-best-leg-strengthening-exercises-for-seniors

Laferrara, T. (2022, July 11). Work Your Glutes and Thighs With the Dumbbell Lunge. Verywell Fit. https://www.verywellfit.com/how-to-do-dumbbell-lunges-3498297

Lefkowith, C. (2015, July 22). 20 Partner Exercises | Redefining Strength. Redefining Strength. https://redefiningstrength.com/try-these-20-partner-exercises-for-a-fun-full-body-workout/

MasterClass. (2021, June 7). Step-up Exercise Guide: How to Do Step-ups With Perfect Form. MasterClass. https://www.masterclass.com/articles/step-ups-exercise-guide

Medicine Ball Exercises for Seniors | Westwind House. (2019, May 7). West Wind House. https://westwindhouse.com/2019/05/07/medicine-ball-exercises-for-seniors/

Merriam-Webster. (2022). Merriam-Webster Dictionary. Merriam-Webster.com; Merriam-Webster. https://www.merriam-webster.com/

Ogle, M. (2021, August 20). Glutes, Hamstrings, and Why You Need Hip Extension Exercises. Verywell Fit. https://www.verywellfit.com/hip-extension-basics-2704334

Pruznick, M. (n.d.). 4 Tips for Seniors to Maintain and Improve Balance. Wellness.nifs.org. https://wellness.nifs.org/blog/4-tips-for-seniors-to-maintain-and-improve-balance

Robinson, L. (2019). HelpGuide.org. HelpGuide.org. https://www.helpguide.org/articles/healthy-living/exercise-and-fitness-as-you-age.htm

Schrift, D. (n.d.). 12 Best Shoulder Exercises For Seniors And The Elderly – ELDERGYM®. ElderGym. https://eldergym.com/shoulder-exercises/

Schultz, R. (2019, May 10). This Single Move Targets Your Butt, Legs, AND Core. Women's Health. https://www.womenshealthmag.com/fitness/a27423100/single-leg-deadlift-exercise/

Seated vs Standing Exercise. (2016, May 18). Sunwarrior. https://sunwarrior.com/

blogs/health-hub/seated-vs-standing-exercise

Should You Try Resistance Bands for Strength Training? (2019, October 25). Health Essentials from Cleveland Clinic. https://health.clevelandclinic.org/should-you-try-resistance-bands-for-strength-training/

Sikana English. (n.d.-a). Back Exercises with a Partner | Exercise for Older Adults. Www.youtube.com. https://youtu.be/PQGPa3OJ1xg

Sikana English. (n.d.-b). Neck Workouts with a Partner | Exercise for Older Adults. Www.youtube.com. https://www.youtube.com/watch?v=JIKdHAAfnuY

Simpson, L. (2012, November 1). The Importance of Safe Exercise. Www.avenidapartners.com. https://www.avenidapartners.com/blog/the-importance-of-safe-exercise

Stannah. (2020, May 21). The science behind functional Balance: recovering from loss of balance | Stannah. Blog Australia. https://blog.stannah.com.au/health/functional-balance-improve-sense-of-balance/

Street Parking. (n.d.). 6 Benefits of Using Dumbbells in Your Workouts. Street Parking. https://streetparking.com/blogs/news/6-benefits-of-using-dumbbells-in-your-workouts

Test Your Balance With Balance Tests. (2018, January 24). BetterPT Blog. https://www.betterpt.com/post/test-your-balance-with-balance-tests

The 7 Best Dumbbell Exercises to Boost Senior's Power. (2021, May 15). Living Maples. https://livingmaples.com/mag/dumbbell-exercises-for-elderly

The Importance of Being Balanced | Preventous Collaborative Health. (2010, August 27). Preventous Collaborative Health | Calgary Private Medical Clinic. https://preventous.com/the-importance-of-being-balanced/

Thiamwong, L., & Suwanno, J. (2014). Effects of Simple Balance Training on Balance Performance and Fear of Falling in Rural Older Adults. International Journal of Gerontology, 8(3), 143–146. https://doi.org/10.1016/j.ijge.2013.08.011

Very Well Fit. (2019). Beginner Ball Workout for Balance, Stability, and Core Strength. Verywell Fit. https://www.verywellfit.com/ball-workout-for-balance-and-strength-1230908

Vestibular Rehabilitation. (2018, May 4). Cleveland Clinic. https://my.clevelandclinic.org/health/treatments/15298-vestibular-rehabilitation

Vestibular_Exercises. (n.d.). University of Mississippi Medical Center. https://www.umc.edu/Healthcare/ENT/Patient-Handouts/Adult/Otology/Vestibular_Exercises.html

Watson, S. (2020, November 23). Balance Training: Benefits, Intensity Level, and More. WebMD. https://www.webmd.com/fitness-exercise/a-z/balance-training#:~:text=Balance%20training%20involves%20doing%20exercises

Williams, L. (2022, July 26). Toast Your Quads and Build Your Butt With the Bulgarian Split Squat. Verywell Fit. https://www.verywellfit.com/how-to-do-a-bulgarian-split-squat-4589307

Yoga Side-bending Poses for Beginners. (2015, April 12). EverydayYoga.com. https://www.everydayyoga.com/blogs/guides/yoga-side-bending-poses-for-beginners

Zlatopolsky, A. (2022, July 1). 6 Unexpected Health Benefits of Walking—Plus How to Make This Underrated Exercise a Habit. Real Simple. https://www.realsimple.com/health/fitness-exercise/walking-benefits

Printed in Great Britain
by Amazon